Clearing the Path

Clearing the Path

On Death, Loss, and Grief

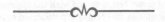

Lynne Dale Halamish, MA, CT

*Thanatologist: Lecturer, Trainer and Counselor on
Death and Dying, Loss and Grieving,
Member of the Kappy and Eric Flanders National Palliative Care
Resource Centre of Ben Gurion University of the Negev, Israel*

With contribution from Eric J. Cassell, MD, MACP

*Emeritus Professor of Public Health,
Weill Medical College of Cornell University;
Adjunct Professor of Medicine,
Faculty of Medicine, McGill University;
Attending Physician at the NewYork-Presbyterian Hospital;
Adjunct Professor of Medical Humanities, Baylor University, Texas*

OXFORD
UNIVERSITY PRESS

OXFORD
UNIVERSITY PRESS

Oxford University Press is a department of the University of Oxford. It furthers
the University's objective of excellence in research, scholarship, and education
by publishing worldwide. Oxford is a registered trade mark of Oxford University
Press in the UK and certain other countries.

Published in the United States of America by Oxford University Press
198 Madison Avenue, New York, NY 10016, United States of America.

Library of Congress Cataloging-in-Publication Data
Names: Halamish, Lynne Dale, author. | Cassell, Eric J., 1928-2021, author.
Title: Clearing the path : on death, loss, and grief / Lynne Dale Halamish
with Eric J. Cassell.
Description: New York, NY : Oxford University Press, [2022] |
Includes bibliographical references and index.
Identifiers: LCCN 2021051189 (print) | LCCN 2021051190 (ebook) |
ISBN 9780197636879 (paperback) | ISBN 9780197636893 (epub) |
ISBN 9780197636909
Subjects: MESH: Attitude to Death | Grief | Terminal Care | Family
Relations | Terminally Ill—psychology | Adaptation, Psychological
Classification: LCC BF789.D4 (print) | LCC BF789.D4 (ebook) | NLM BF
789.D4 | DDC 155.9/37—dc23/eng/20211124
LC record available at https://lccn.loc.gov/2021051189
LC ebook record available at https://lccn.loc.gov/2021051190

DOI: 10.1093/oso/9780197636879.001.0001

This material is not intended to be, and should not be considered, a substitute for medical or
other professional advice. Treatment for the conditions described in this material is highly
dependent on the individual circumstances. And, while this material is designed to offer accurate
information with respect to the subject matter covered and to be current as of the time it was
written, research and knowledge about medical and health issues is constantly evolving and
dose schedules for medications are being revised continually, with new side effects recognized
and accounted for regularly. Readers must therefore always check the product information and
clinical procedures with the most up-to-date published product information and data sheets
provided by the manufacturers and the most recent codes of conduct and safety regulation.
The publisher and the authors make no representations or warranties to readers, express or
implied, as to the accuracy or completeness of this material. Without limiting the foregoing, the
publisher and the authors make no representations or warranties as to the accuracy or efficacy
of the drug dosages mentioned in the material. The authors and the publisher do not accept,
and expressly disclaim, any responsibility for any liability, loss, or risk that may be claimed or
incurred as a consequence of the use and/or application of any of the contents of this material.

1 3 5 7 9 8 6 4 2
Printed by Marquis, Canada

"Yea, though I walk through the valley of the shadow of death . . ."
For El Elyon

CONTENTS

PREFACE

Clearing the Path: On Death, Loss, and Grief is a collection of true stories from the field. As with its companion volume, *The Weeping Willow: Encounters with Grief*, real-life parables are employed to illustrate practical communication tools, which can be applied by both the caregivers and the recipients of that care: dying patients and/or grievers.

Also like the previous book, the distinguishing features of *Clearing the Path* are its brevity and clarity. Although many other firsthand clinical reports supply the advice found here, the storytelling style we chose has the advantage of providing something more: a glimpse into the authentic human emotions experienced by both counselors and clients in these typical and atypical encounters with dying and grieving.

This book, written 13 years after *The Weeping Willow*, presents more complex encounters and more nuanced emotions, drawn from those additional years of experience in the field. And because we learn more about ourselves from every new encounter, this experience has deepened that self-knowledge, along with appreciation for its teaching value. Thus, these new stories allow the reader to share several "Aha!" moments in my practice, as I, myself, experienced them.

The book's primary audience includes medical practitioners, nursing staff, psychotherapists, social workers, counselors, chaplains or other pastoral care providers, researchers, and gerontologists who work in both hospital and home-care settings. *Clearing the Path* can benefit professionals at all levels of experience, even serving as textbook instruction for clinical training programs in healthcare or psychosocial practice. In keeping with that focus, each story is followed by a section designated as Notes to the Practitioner.

However, *Clearing the Path* is also practical for patients and their families who are coming to terms with a terminal illness, preparing to have difficult end-of-life conversations, or coping with grief after a death.

Each chapter in *Clearing the Path* contains a vignette, with teaching notes frequently embedded in the story as "aside" comments. The chapters are an average of one to five pages long. They are followed by Notes to the Practitioner, where we try to pinpoint the most essential challenges and lessons in each story, so that they can be added to your communication repertoire. The Notes are followed by Conclusions, a section summarizing the chapter message(s) in a few main points; and Recommended Readings, additional reading for those who would like to pursue that topic further.

Some readers may be hoping that *Clearing the Path* offers detailed, skills-based information on preparing for difficult conversations, such as the appropriate words to use and/or the theory behind each strategy. This is not a "how-to" book in that conventional sense. Instead, it teaches by examples gleaned from hands-on counseling experience. That said, the Notes to the Practitioner are meant to specifically address preparedness for common end-of-life situations with professional directives, further reinforced by the Conclusions and Recommended Readings.

We are teachers. But although we teach by lecturing, counseling, supervision, and writing, we believe teaching by example, through stories from the field, is a very effective tool.

That acknowledgment recognizes that communication is individual and that it's dependent on all the involved parties. Thus, the stories were selected to demonstrate many ways of communication through a range of situations, as well as the various attitudes (helpful and hurtful) revealed in responses from people surrounding the patient and/or griever. However, despite the differences between people and stories, there are common denominators that make these tools highly applicable in many circumstances.

DISCLAIMER

A counselor first needs to understand the client's or patient's belief system, to work within that worldview. This is not limited to religious faith but involves a core of individual beliefs (and cultural taboos) regarding the proper limits of healthcare, the point at which life ends, what death brings, how to part from the living, and how to honor the dead—to name a few.

The only certainty is that there is no such thing as a tabula rasa, a blank slate, regarding questions of life and death. Counselors *always* bring themselves into the interchange, whether or not they choose to recognize it.

During my years of practice, I have worked from a very clearly defined belief system. I believe in God as the Creator and Ruler of the universe.

I believe that all humans are made in God's image, and as such they deserve mercy, care, and respect. As I illustrated throughout both books, I ask questions to clarify the life-and-death beliefs held by each of them. I don't argue with my clients, regardless of their belief system, unless I have reason to think they may be a threat to themselves or to others.

WARNING

If you are working in the field of death and dying, grieving and loss, even part-time, *please* be careful. Do not drown in it. Remember what is yours to carry, and what is not. Allow yourself time to heal from your work, and from any other issues you may be facing.

As always in teaching, as well as in writing, we leave you with the blessing of Jonathan Swift, "May you live every day of your life."

ACKNOWLEDGMENTS

I would like to express sincere thanks to:

All of the people who generously allowed us to use their stories, so that we could teach/help others to recover from loss. Without them, this book would not exist.

Eric J. Cassell, who believed in this project, this work, and this vision; who walked through every word; whose presence is felt throughout my work; and who generously agreed to be part of this endeavor.

Hilah Mazyar, first editor, for creative titles, wisdom, and support throughout the project.

Hannah Weiss, final editor, dear friend, and wise woman, for invaluable accurate feedback and editing.

Michael Hillel, for valuable and important research.

Toni Schulke, for helping to resolve points of confusion in this book.

Oxford University Press, especially Marta Moldovi, for clear and timely guidance, Tiffany Lu, for initiating this second book and Sujitha Logagansan, for clarity and patience.

To my amazing family: Asaf, Shachar, Hilah, and Oriah, for their unstinting support, love, and willingness to be exposed where I exposed myself. To Zohar, who walks with us.

To my siblings: Toni, Jordan, Rachel, Naomi, and Rachelli, for their support and encouragement.

To Yoram Singer, for insightful feedback and contributions to this book.

To Sivan Fiterman, for the beautiful artwork on the cover.

And primarily, to the one true God, Creator of heaven and earth, for every breath we take, who guides us if we take His hand, and whose mercies are new every morning.

GRIEF MAP

This is a "Road Map of Grief." It is designed to help you find your way around if you don't want to read the entire book and are looking for practical tools to deal with a specific situation.

HOW TO USE THE MAP

1. In the top row, find the relationship that is the subject of your concern.
2. In the left-hand column, find the specific issue that concerns you.
3. The intersection of these two items will direct you to the relevant chapter(s).
4. Chapters are indicated either numerically or with A or B for the appendixes.

Grief Map		Children	Teenagers/ Young adults	Parents
Issue of concern	Lingering Death	2,8,11,	2	1,2,3,8,9,
	Sudden Death			12,16,29,30
	Funeral	8,13,24,	8	8,12,
	Grief Rituals	13,24,A,B	15	12,16,
	Repercussions of Loss		15,17	16,29,30
	Length of Grief		15	16
	Returning to Life after Loss	8	15	8,16,29,30
	Transference			
	Body Language	2, 24, 17,	2,17	1,2,12,16,
	Suicidal Intent/suicide		16	16
	Moment of Death			3,
	Truth Telling	2,8,10,13,17	17	1,2,8,11,16,29
	Practical Solutions	10,8,11,17,24,A	15,17,20,A	1,2,8,11,12,16,30,A
	Perception and Language	10,8,17,24	17	29
	Listening	8,10,24,A		2,8,12,16,29
	Cost vs Benefit	8,	1	1,8,12,30
	Talking about Death	2,8,10,11,17,24,A,B	1,2,15,17	1,2,3,8,11,12,16
	Preparation for Death	2,8,11,13	1,2,	1,2,3,8,11,
	Decision Making	2,8,	2,20,	1,2,8,12,16
	Saying Goodbye	8,9,11,24	1	1,8,9,11,12,16
	Hope			16,29,30
	End of Grief	B	15,B	16,30,B
	Looking for Meaning	5,9,11,13,24	20	5,9,12,16,29,30
	Silence	24		16

Grief Map

Widows/ers	Professionals	Dying/seriously ill person	Adults/Partners
	2,3,22,A	1,2,3,4,5,6,9,11,13,	1,2,3,9,22,
18,19,23	12,23		
	12, A	13,14	14
18,19,	A,B		17
18,19,23,A,B	20,23,B	25,27	17, 28,
	B		17
18,19,23,A,B	12,21,23,30,B	27	17, 28
	20,21,22		22,
18,26,A	2,3,10,22,23	1,2,3,14,25	1,3,14,17,22,26,28
19,26		25	26
A,B	3,A,B	3,7,	3,
18,19,23	1,3,7,10,20,21,23,A,B	1,2,3,4,5,6,9,13,25,27,	1,2,3,9,17,
18,19,A	1,2,3,7,8,10,12,21,23,A,B	1,2,3,5,7,9,11,13,14,27	3,14,17,28
18,23,A,B	20,21,22,B	5,9, 14,25,	9,14,17,22,
18,19,23,A,B	1,2,3,5,7,10,12,21,22,A,B	1,2,3,5,7,13,14,25,	1,2,3,9,14,17,22,28,
	20	1,6,7, 11,13,25,27,	1,
18,19,23	1,2,3,7,10, 12,23,A	1,2,3,4,7,9,11,13,14,25,	1,2,3,9,14,17,
	1,2,3,7,A	1,2,3,7,9,11,13,14,	1,2,3,9,14,
18,19,23	20	1,2,9,11,14,25,27,	1,2,9,14,17,28,
19,A	7,9,	1,6,7,9,11,14,	1,9,14,
18,19,23		4,7,25,27,	17,28,30,B
19,B	23,30,B		B
19,23	7,12,22	4,6,9,11,13,14,25	14,17,28
19	1,5,A,B	25	17,A,B

I

———⊶⊷———

Preparing for Death

1

⌇⌇

Living Eulogy

Giving the Patient Maximum Control

I was flown in by the Health Committee of the small town. They wanted me to meet with a family in distress. They felt the family, who was well loved in their town, was in turmoil while facing the impending death of the father.

Right off the plane, I was brought to the patient's private hospital room.

The father of the family, Benny, aged 64, was dying of cancer.

I was told that neither his family nor he recognized that he was dying. The battle was already lost, according to the health professionals. Yet the family wanted to keep fighting for his life in every possible way.

I walked into a room full of blotchy-faced people who had obviously been crying. A gaunt man took up the middle portion of the hospital bed, which looked a lot larger due to his small size.

I introduced myself briefly and then asked to be introduced to those in the room. I met Benny, who took my hand as I introduced myself; followed by Benny's wife Janet, and their three children: Eve (32), Joseph (28), and Dave (23).

Janet and Benny lived in the family home with their youngest, Dave, and Janet's mother, Roma, to whom Janet was very close.

They told me that Roma was "driving Benny crazy." However, due to Janet's close relationship with her mother, I knew that she would be a much-needed lifeline for Janet after Benny's death.

Clearing the Path. Lynne Dale Halamish and Eric J. Cassell, Oxford University Press. © Lynne Dale Halamish 2022.
DOI: 10.1093/oso/9780197636879.003.0001

I briefly sketched out a genogram to keep the names, ages, and family positions straight in my own mind. I showed the family what I was doing as I wrote.

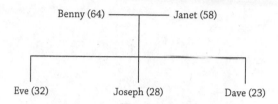

Benny was lying in bed; his skin had a distinct yellow color. He seemed very weak. He had a lot of extra skin around his jaw and neck, indicating that he had lost a considerable amount of weight. His eyes were at half-mast and frequently closed—I assumed this was due to the morphine. However, although interspersed with long pauses, his answers to all questions were clear and full of intent.

He spoke with difficulty, frequently asking for water or gel to moisten his mouth. His daughter, Eve, would help him with the gel, wearing a disposable glove and massaging it into his mouth periodically. His youngest, Dave, would bring him water. Occasionally, three or four family members would adjust Benny's position by pulling his cover sheet back to move him into a more comfortable angle in bed.

"Are you in pain?," I asked.

"It's manageable," he answered.

I asked for more details about his illness. After listening intently for several minutes, I finally asked, "So, Benny . . . What is going to happen?"

"The disease has won," he replied plainly.

Whoever explained this situation to Benny has done a good job, I thought to myself. But I still wanted to make sure he understood. "What do you mean?"

He answered simply, "The end."

There was silence between us as we regarded each other. We could both hear the sniffles of some of Benny's family members after hearing his answers.

"What is the hardest thing about the end for you?" I continued, never taking my eyes away from him.

"I don't know how it's going to be."

"I see," I answered, and remained quiet for about a minute before going on. To many people, this lack of knowledge can be very frightening.

Most people have never witnessed a death, and it is full of unknowns. In the disorienting journey of terminal illness, even knowing that it will most likely be hard gives a sense of more control than not knowing even that much.

"Are you having any lung issues? How is your breathing?"

"It's okay. My lungs are fine."

"In that case, it will probably be okay. You will not be gasping for air. You will spend more and more time sleeping, and then, most likely, you will lose consciousness. You need to ask your physician, because I am not familiar with all the aspects of your condition, but I think if you ask calmly, he will answer."

I glanced at the other family members who were silently witnessing our exchange, some still weeping, others looking concerned or exhausted.

"Is there anything after death, Benny?"

In order to understand the person I am working with when dealing with imminent death, this question is important.

"I don't know. I don't think so."

I looked around the room. "Who makes the decisions about Benny's medical condition?"

Joseph answered, "The family."

"That is not an answer," I said. "Which member of the family makes the necessary decisions?" I reiterated.

Joseph again answered, "We all do."

"No, you all don't," I replied quietly. "Who is the one who actually decides?"

"Mom does," said someone. ". . . But she consults us first."

"She can consult whomever she wishes, but is the final word hers?" I turned to Janet for confirmation. "Do you make the decisions?"

"Yes," she replied quietly, her eyes meeting mine.

I turned to Benny. "Why don't *you* make the decisions, Benny?"

There is frequently a tendency to relate to seriously ill people like children, making decisions for them even when they are capable of making them for themselves. This takes away the fragile grip that they had on any remaining sense of control.

I slowly looked around the room to address the entire family.

"I know Benny's illness and the threat to his life affect you all very profoundly. However, it's still Benny's life. It's Benny's body, and it's Benny's death. He should be making the decisions. Unless he doesn't want to."

Silence.

I turned back to the dying man.

"Benny, do you want to make the decisions about your body?"

"Yes."

"So, what do *you* want?"

"I don't want to be hooked up to any machines. And . . . And I don't want to be resuscitated if I lose consciousness."

I looked around the room once again.

"Did everyone hear that?" They nodded. "So, what will you all do?"

Several of them responded together. "We won't resuscitate him, and we won't hook him up to any machines." There were many tears on many faces at this point.

"Benny has given you a wonderful gift. He has decided. He has taken responsibility. That means you don't have to decide for him. That means no guilt."

Then I turned to him. "Benny, you are free to change your mind at any point, if you want to. If you don't change your mind, we will assume what you have just said is what you want. Is that right?"

"Yes." His voice was faint but steady.

"Benny, is there anything else you would like?" I asked him.

Benny added that he wanted to be moved to a teaching hospice, so that as he dies, he can help advance the research on his disease and perhaps help others who are suffering with it. This shocked and worried his family. They said they never suspected he would want something like that.

Clarification: Revealing unexpected wishes like this is one of the important aspects of meeting the whole family together with the patient.

During this time, various family members said things. Everyone contributed—except for Dave, who sat right next to Benny but did not speak, except through occasional grunts of assent.

I began the next topic this way: "Benny, tell me a little about yourself. What kind of a man are you? What is important to you?"

He shifted in his bed. "Well, I am not an easy man. I have a lot of expectations."

"From yourself, or others?" I asked.

"Both."

His family chimed in: "He knows what he wants, and he gets it."

I turned to his wife with a half-smile. "Did that include getting you?"

The family laughed, and Janet told me the story of their courtship.

Benny then told me about his work throughout his life, his dedication to his country and fellow man, and his drive to improve things for his community. His family also took part in this discussion.

I observed, "You all sound very proud of your father; and you, Janet, of your husband."

This forum allows Benny to hear his eulogy without naming it as such. It is good for him to hear about his impact on the community and his family while he is still alive and conscious. It's also an opportunity to reminisce and laugh together as a family. Additionally, it helps ease the tension a bit, as a break from the painful subjects we were discussing.

The responses were pouring out from several directions at once. "Dad is a great man. He has done so much. He is well loved by everyone, both for his personality and for his high expectations. People try to live up to his expectations and become better for it."

"Do you do this, too?" I asked his children.

"Yes!" they all answered . . . Except for Dave, who held his peace.

It is worth mentioning that throughout our meeting, I shifted back and forth between Benny's past and present. It is difficult to maintain concentration if we only stay on difficult subjects. If they are interspersed with memories, analysis, and even introspection ("What do you think made you that way?"), there are many benefits to be gained: recognizing who Benny has been, indulging in a little comic relief, recognizing each family member by commenting on something I can observe about them, and improving their concentration for the decisions that need to be made now.

After a while, we returned to the subject of death.

"Benny, what frightens you about death?"

"Lack of control."

In acknowledgment, I preserved a few moments of silence before continuing.

"If you tell us what you want, Benny, we will respect your wishes, as much as it is in our power."

This is an opportunity for the caregiver to clarify his or her limitations. For example: "We will not do anything illegal"; "We cannot provide for someone who needs an IV in his own home"; "We do not perform assisted suicide"; "If you require special supportive furniture and wide doorways, and this isn't available in your home, we cannot send you home"; and so forth.

A tool I like to use at this point is the set of "Go Wish" cards (http://www.gowish.org). Even professionals who frequently work in this field can forget to ask the relevant questions. These cards lay out the issues clearly, giving the dying person a wide range of choices about the period prior to the end of life. I showed Benny the cards and explained how they work. We went through them.

"Does this feel more like control?" I asked him.

"Yes, it does," he answered.

It was time for the family's role to be recognized. "I know it is very hard for you to hear that the disease has won. To know that your time together is limited. What will you do with the time you have left?"

They replied as a chorus: "We will be with him as much as we can. We will laugh with him, and we will not leave him alone."

I pointed out their advantage. "You know, with this terrible disease comes a wonderful opportunity. You have some time. Time to *really* communicate. Not like a car accident, where—bang—and it's over. *Use* the time you have. It is a gift."

I went on to explain the Five Things (see Recommended Reading no. 2) necessary for saying goodbye to a dying loved one (see Chapter 19) "Forgive me," "I forgive you," "I love you," "Thank you," and "Goodbye". I also gave them ground rules:

"The Five Things are private. It is not a family activity. One-on-one only. If you do it in a group, the chances of honesty are slim . . . Everyone will be tempted to cover up things."

"You are racing the clock. Do this today or tomorrow. Do *not* put it off. Not because Benny will die today or tomorrow," I smiled at him, "but because this door does not close when Benny dies. It closes when communication with him is no longer possible. Communication can stop because of the disease, or the treatment, or because of pain or fatigue. *There is no time to spare.*"

I turned to Benny. "Benny, you have a harder job than anyone else in this room, because each one only has to tell these five things to you, but you have to tell them to each of the four members of your family. Can you do that, Benny?"

His gaze reflected his determination. "I will do it."

I was able to get a ride back to my hotel with Dave, the silent son. Following my meeting with the family, his mother had told me that Dave hadn't spoken to anyone about Benny's worsening condition. Janet believed that I should try to get him to talk. It was the same directive I had received from the staff about Dave before my visit.

I wasn't sure that this was a good strategy. It is true that most people benefit from talking about their feelings, but not everyone does.

I sat quietly in the passenger seat while Dave drove us. After a while, I asked, "Dave, are you more like your mom or your dad?"

He smiled as he answered. "Everyone tells me I am *exactly* like my dad." And he arched an eyebrow at the road in front of him for emphasis.

"Is that good or bad?"

"Both," he replied with a wry grin.

We were again silent for several minutes. It seemed to me to be a comfortable silence. I wasn't sure that Dave, who had lived with his father and frequently cared for his physical needs, could verbalize his devotion. He needed to hear that wordless love is also acceptable.

I began, "Dave, you know, there are many languages of love." I paused. "Sometimes it's in words, but many times our language is expressed in actions. Sometimes, words can even be unnecessary."

I waited a few moments before asking him what would be the hardest thing for him about losing his father.

He replied, "He won't be there for things in my life."

I responded, "Yes, that is very hard. You are the youngest and will have had him for the shortest time. It's very hard. It makes *this* time all the more important."

The next morning, I was informed that each family member, including Dave, had already had private time with Benny to say the Five Things. And he had done the same with each of them.

Benny had been uncommunicative for days before my visit. No one was sure if he would be able to talk with me. In the end, we spoke for two and a half hours, and Benny was very coherent throughout the entire time. And during the one-on-one talks with each of his family members, he managed to stay focused for even longer than that.

The day after those private talks, he was uncommunicative again. He had rallied himself expressly for the meetings and then lapsed into a coma.

Three days later, Benny died, never having regained consciousness.

NOTES TO THE PRACTITIONER

This case illustrates the importance of family communication and consensus with the dying patient. Initially, the practitioners must clarify for themselves what the patient and family actually know. This is also a way to discover misconceptions and correct them where necessary.

Because of the helplessness or feelings of loss of control that terminal illness engenders, it is wise for the staff to give the patient as much control as possible—a kind of dignity maintenance. That is, unless the patient does not want control; in which case, the patient should appoint an individual to whom he or she would like to assign control.

Patients frequently find the "living eulogy" described in this case useful and encouraging. It also has the additional boon of encouraging family members to express things they may not have otherwise expressed to the dying family member, thereby reducing the number of "I wish I had told him . . ." feelings following the death.

Asking the patient to tell his life story is also a very strong message that you, as a health professional, are interested in him not merely as a medical case but also as a human being. This also can increase trust and therefore compliance to your recommendations. For the practitioner, listening to life stories can increase work satisfaction and reduce burnout. Not uncommonly, it improves diagnostic skills and consequently health outcomes.

As explained in the text, switching between difficult topics (such as illness, death, and scary decisions) and lighter observations or shared stories improves patient and family concentration. It also has the added benefit of bringing the family together towards the end of their loved one's life.

CONCLUSIONS

- *Verify any information you are given about the patient or family before you accept it.*
- *Provide maximum control to the patient unless he or she indicates otherwise.*
- *Give permission for the griever to part in his or her own way.*
- *Encourage a eulogy while the patient is still conscious.*
- *Shift subjects, in order to acknowledge the life of the patient, improve concentration, and relieve tension.*

RECOMMENDED READING

1. Marie Curie, "Care and Support through Terminal Illness: Talking to Someone about Dying," February 2021, https://www.mariecurie.org.uk/professionals/palliative-care-knowledge-zone/individual-needs/talking-approaching-end-life (accessed July 26, 2021).
2. Ira Byock, *Dying Well* (New York: Penguin Putnam, 1998).

2

✣

No-Man's Land

Last-Wishes Dilemma

I sat with the two of them at the dining-room table. I asked Dani where she
would like to die. She leaned towards me. "At home," she replied.

I turned to face them both as I responded. "Before you make a final decision about this, you need to know what the death will look like. I don't
have enough knowledge about all aspects of your disease to say for sure.
Ask your physician what it will look like. If you ask him calmly, he should
give you a good idea of what to expect. It might let you regain a sense of
control."

"But," and here I turned to Dani, "if you'd rather not hear it, your husband Natan can hear it for you both." I nodded at him.

She looked down at her hands on the table and repeated, "I really want
to die at home."

I answered quietly, "I understand. But you need to know if your family
can bear it. You have children at home. Even more so, you need to decide
whether you trust Natan to decide what the house, the children, and he
himself can bear when you are no longer conscious."

"Can you trust Natan to do that?" I asked, looking directly into her eyes.

Dani and Natan looked at each other. They didn't speak, but the question was on the table between them. It was clear that they would discuss
this privately.

Five weeks later, Dani lost consciousness. She was in no visible distress
or pain; every line on her face had relaxed. The children, aged 17, 13, and

Clearing the Path. Lynne Dale Halamish and Eric J. Cassell, Oxford University Press. © Lynne Dale Halamish 2022.
DOI: 10.1093/oso/9780197636879.003.0002

8, were told that medicine could no longer provide solutions for her; their mother was dying.

During that time period, all of the children spent less and less time at home. Natan remained by his wife's side. But he was not alone. The house was filled with people coming and going: friends, well-wishers, and medical and mental health personnel.

One evening, Natan sat with the children and asked them, "Would it be okay with you if Mom dies here at home, or would you rather she didn't?" All three of them asked that she not die at home.

"What will I do now?" Natan said to me. "It's not that her upcoming death will be violent or horrific. It's likely to be quiet and peaceful. Yet they all asked that it not happen at home—a place for life, and where their own lives must carry on."

Last wishes have an incredibly strong presence and are very hard for loved ones to defy. However, dying at home can change the associations of the place for the surviving family members. Instead of being life-giving and nurturing, the home can be seen as a dangerous, uncomfortable, or unclean place.

The decision was Natan's. He told the children that in the morning they would move their mom to the nursing facility just down the road from their home. While still feeling torn between Dani's last wishes and their children's wishes, he arranged the time for the ambulance to come. In the process, he did not even know or ask what his own wishes were.

In the morning, the ambulance arrived to move Dani to the nursing facility, where she did *not* want to die.

She was gently and respectfully arranged on the ambulance gurney. The paramedics raised the gurney into the ambulance. Natan climbed in to sit beside her, and the doors closed behind him. He reached out and gently touched Dani's arm.

As the engine started and they began to move, Dani took her final breath. She didn't die at home, and she didn't die in the nursing facility.

"Thank you," Natan whispered to the lifeless form beside him.

NOTES TO THE PRACTITIONER

Last wishes can be problematic, but not knowing what those last wishes are can be even more detrimental. If, for example, Dani had not been asked where she would like to die, the family would never have known what she wanted.

We may be tempted not to ask the patient about last wishes, fearful that perhaps we cannot grant them. In this case, the problem with granting Dani's wish was becoming apparent as her death approached. The children began spending less and less time at home, because it became a place that no longer belonged exclusively to the immediate family. It no longer felt safe to the children.

The home belongs to the survivors of a death. As such, it must remain a safe, life-giving place for them. It was clear that Dani's concern for her children was paramount throughout her life and illness. Therefore, when they made their request that she not die in the home, according to everything we know about her, she would have chosen to leave.

We can never know in advance what changes in the situation may occur in real time. In case the dying person's last wishes cannot be granted, it's important to include an escape clause: "Do you trust your loved ones to make the right decision when the time comes?"

I would like to clarify here that this decision, whether or not to die in the home, can vary according to family and relationship. Sometimes a peaceful death at home is very comforting to the survivors. But sometimes it is not . . . and for this reason, we need to ask.

If at all possible, have all family members present during any "last wishes" discussion. Sometimes, for various reasons, this is not an option. But it is worthwhile to make the attempt.

CONCLUSIONS

- *Last wishes are important, even when they cannot be granted. If the last wishes are either illegal or impractical, that needs to be discussed and clarified with the patient.*
- *The other option, in this case, was not to ask the children. However, this does not change what the children experience; it only hides it from those who should be protecting them.*
- *The conclusion here is not that the patient should die at home or somewhere else, but rather to find out what the patient's wishes are, what the family wishes are, and help to make a decision that is appropriate for both.*

RECOMMENDED READING

1. *JAMA Internal Medicine* 173(13) (July 8, 2013): 1241–1245, doi:10.1001/jamainternmed.2013.6053.

2.   L. A. Roscoe, "Being Clear about Your Last Wishes Can Make Death Easier for You and Loved Ones," May 2018, https://theconversation.com/being-clear-about-your-last-wishes-can-make-death-easier-for-you-and-loved-ones-95345 (accessed July 26, 2021).

3.   Josee-Lyne Ethier, Thivaher Paramsothy, John J. You et al., "Perceived Barriers to Goals of Care Discussions with Patients with Advanced Cancer and Their Families in the Ambulatory Setting: A Multicenter Survey of Oncologists," *Sage Journal of Palliative Care* 33(3) (April 2018), https://doi.org/10.1177/08258 59718762287 (accessed July 26, 2021).

3

⌘

Ready When You Are

Preparing for Death

When do patients and/or their families know that they, or their loved ones, are dying?

There are two correct answers to this question:

1. They always know.
2. They never know.

The difference between knowing something on an intellectual level and knowing something on an emotional level is vast. In this respect, dying is the same as being bereaved: you know that it will happen, you see it coming, you talk about it, you prepare for it . . . and when it actually happens, you can't believe it.

I received a call from Tami and her husband, Marcus. They told me that Tami was dying, and they wanted a consultation at their home. Since their home was a two-hour drive away, I told them that we would have only one meeting.

When I arrived on the agreed day, I saw a couple in their early 70s who seemed very connected and respectful towards each other. Tami was lying in bed in a homey, comfortable room softly illuminated with large windows. Marcus sat in an armchair by her side.

Marcus was Tami's primary caretaker. He cared for her physical needs, did the laundry, cleaned the house, cooked their simple meals, and kept the

Clearing the Path. Lynne Dale Halamish and Eric J. Cassell, Oxford University Press. © Lynne Dale Halamish 2022.
DOI: 10.1093/oso/9780197636879.003.0003

garden green. Thanks to the large bedroom windows, she was never out of his sight.

"Tami only has the strength to speak for about 20 minutes," Marcus had warned me at the beginning of our meeting. Nevertheless, the three of us spoke for two and a half hours.

It was clear that both of them had prepared very well for my one-time visit. I began by asking Marcus how he was coping.

"Are you eating, Marcus? Have you lost any weight recently? How have you been sleeping? Do you have any time off from taking care of Tami?"

This line of questioning seemed to surprise them both. Marcus answered my questions, and he added, "I'm happy to be here, and I'm glad that I retired just in time to care for Tami."

During our time together, their hands often reached for each other, and their fingers would intertwine during the more difficult parts. Their eyes often met with tender compassion, periodically glistening with tears. They sporadically smiled at one another. Tami would pet Marcus's head now and then as he sighed.

Then, we spoke about saying goodbye: when, to whom, where, and how. It was like several weeks of meetings compressed into one.

I thought that they were probably concerned about how the end would come. I asked her: "Tami, would you like to know how your death will most likely occur?"

Rather than being startled by my question, both of them looked relieved. "Yes, very much," Tami replied, and Marcus nodded in agreement. He stood up, got a pad of paper and a pen, resumed his seat and looked at me, waiting for me to speak.

I went on to describe the most likely scenario, given the specifics of her physical condition. We spoke about how Tami would physically respond, what her husband would see, the things that may bother them both, and how best to deal with them.

"Tami's pain can be managed." I smiled at her briefly. "You have been working with excellent home-hospice physicians. Your disease does not affect your lungs or throat, and so with reasonable assurance, we can predict how you will die."

I momentarily paused to let them absorb my words, and then went on. "If nothing changes physically, you will be sleeping more and more, until you finally lose consciousness." I paused again and waited for both sets of eyes to meet mine again, ready for what would follow. They tightened their handclasp.

"Nearing the end . . ." I paused, "you will most likely begin to breathe progressively louder." I went on to describe the abnormal pattern of breathing known as Cheyne-Stokes respiration. Marcus was intently taking notes. He wrote the phrase down on his pad.

"People around you will probably find this disturbing. However, as far as we know, this does not bother the dying person."

"What causes the sound?" Marcus asked.

"It is caused by saliva in the trachea, combined with the body's weakened state. The dying person does not regularly swallow anymore, hence the sound. What this noise does tell us . . . is that the end is likely very near."

I did not try to hurry the conversation. I spoke slowly and clearly, paying close attention to their body language before carrying on. "If the sound is too disturbing, you could gently turn Tami onto her side and place a tissue on the pillow under her mouth. Some of the saliva will drain onto the tissue, which will reduce the noise somewhat."

Turning back to Tami, I went into more detail. "Each breath will come further and further apart, and family members may think that it's over, until another breath is drawn. The very last breath is usually a single, long exhale, which is probably why it is sometimes described as the spirit leaving the body." The three of us sat silently for a time.

"The immediate grief of those present at the time of death usually follows that last exhale. It often begins with a statement like 'It's over now' or 'That's it' or 'She's gone.'"

Again, silence filled the room for several moments.

We then spoke about the family being present at Tami's death, which was what they both wanted.

"Marcus, this will be a tough time, but probably a quiet one. It's also important, if you can, that you pay attention to your grown children and their responses to Tami."

"In what way?" he asked.

"If someone is standing far from the bed and muttering about how she is suffering, when she isn't, gently lead them closer to the bed and point out the relaxed look on her face and lack of tension in her shoulders." I smiled again at Tami, and she returned my smile. "If the family member can see that it's not her pain but their own pain that they're feeling, their memory of the death will be peaceful and serene. If not, they will remember that Tami suffered, even if there was no evidence to support that."

Marcus took his hand off the pad of paper once again to extend his hand to Tami. They both smiled fondly at each other.

"Is there anything else you would like to discuss?" I asked.

Tami replied shyly, "If possible, I would like to maintain my dignity."

"What is dignity, Tami? What do you mean exactly?"

"Well," she continued wistfully, "I would like to be kept clean."

"Okay. Suppose you can no longer control your urine or bowel movements. Would diapers maintain your dignity?"

"Oh, yes, diapers," she replied with unmistakable relief. "That would keep my bed and me clean. Yes, that would be good."

"What else?"

"I don't want my children to act as my caretakers for intimate tasks," she asserted.

"You mean showers and diapers?" Always make sure of what is meant. Never assume.

"Yes."

"Who *should* be the one in charge of performing those intimate tasks?" I inquired.

"Only a nursing aide or Marcus." Those were all the answers I needed from her.

I turned my attention back to Marcus: "Is that acceptable to you?"

"Oh, certainly," he nodded and squeezed Tami's hand warmly with his.

After making sure there were no more questions left unanswered, I left the couple's home, accompanied by their words of gratitude.

Two weeks later, Marcus called and said that Tami had died in a way similar to our discussion. "She said goodbye to each family member, even the young grandchildren, and to some of her close friends. We were ready, and it really was peaceful and serene. Thank you."

I reminded him, "This was a success in saying goodbye. You should rightly feel good about it—you both did well." I paused for a moment.

"Marcus, I want you to be aware that the euphoria you're feeling is temporary. It will soon give way to grief and emptiness. But, Marcus, although it will last a long time, this, too, will be temporary. All grief has a beginning, a middle . . . and the possibility of an end. It's important to understand that reaching the end of grief does not mean erasing or forgetting your loved one."

NOTES TO THE PRACTITIONER

When you first visit a dying person, either in a home-hospice setting, or visiting a dying person in hospital, pay attention to the caretakers. Recognize them as significant. Ask the caretakers how they are coping, whether or not they are eating, sleeping, exercising, and getting some time off from the weight of caring for their loved one who is dying.

Ask the patient and primary caregiver whether or not they would like to know what the end will look and feel like. Most laypeople have never witnessed death, and this unknown can be quite frightening. Check the details of the illness and give a description of what they can expect. Be as specific as you can. But if you are asked a question that you're not sure how to answer, do not guess. Tell them that you will find out and get back to them with an answer.

If any family members are keeping their distance from the dying person, for fear of seeing him suffer, when it is apparent that he is not, bring them closer to the bed and point out visible signs of relaxation in the patient. These can include a relaxed jaw, relaxation between the eyebrows and between the shoulders, and hands that are open rather than clenched. Showing them these signs of ease will help them to remember the death as it was and to understand that the dying patient was not suffering; *the family member* was suffering.

Words like "dignity," "intimate tasks," and "peaceful" can mean different things to different people. Do not guess or try to think what you would want in the patient's place. Try to have the patient define such terms explicitly, so that you can understand what their statement or request really means and what you can do to assist them.

CONCLUSIONS

- *Pay attention not only to your patient but also to the caregiver. Recognize this person.*
- *Advance information about how the death will likely occur, even if difficult, is usually preferable to the unknown.*
- *When a family member "sees" the dying person suffering, where no suffering is apparent, addressing this by pointing out the visible signs of ease will help the family member's memory of the death.*

RECOMMENDED READING

1.   J. Martín Martín, M. Olano-Lizarraga, and M. Saracíbar-Razquin, "The Experience of Family Caregivers Caring for a Terminal Patient at Home: A Research Review," *International Journal of Nursing Studies* 64 (September 2016): 1–12, https://pub med.ncbi.nlm.nih.gov/27657662/ (accessed July 26, 2021).

2.   "A Guide to Understanding End of Life Signs and Symptoms," 2021, https://www.crossroadshospice.com/hospice-resources/end-of-life-signs/ (accessed July 26, 2021).

4

⚭

The Phoenix

Dealing with Recurring Illness and Remissions

Sasha was physically tiny. But as a businesswoman, she was a high-powered bulldozer, at the top of her field (Sales Management for a large international corporation). She had two preschool-aged daughters, and had just given birth to another daughter, when she got the diagnosis: genetically related metastatic breast cancer.

We began to meet immediately after that.

Sasha told me that in the few seconds it took to hear her test results, her world changed beyond recognition. Her established position in the business world, her status, the glamour and air of importance surrounding who she was—it all disappeared in a puff of smoke.

The business world, which she used to see as her battlefield, turned out to have been a walk in the park, compared to the real war she had just entered. Suddenly, all that mattered to her was survival, not for business or reputation, but simply for the privilege of living and raising her three young children.

Sasha entered the new battlefield. She won the first round and went into remission.

Our meetings then centered on reinventing herself. Who should she be now? What should she do with her reclaimed life? She tried to go back to her previous life in the working world, but that world couldn't understand her. Sasha's husband, Simon, didn't get it either. She was well now; where

Clearing the Path. Lynne Dale Halamish and Eric J. Cassell, Oxford University Press. © Lynne Dale Halamish 2022.
DOI: 10.1093/oso/9780197636879.003.0004

was the fireball he had married? Her commitment to her work faded. So we explored other possibilities together.

She took on a more minor role, one with less traveling, to allow for more time with her kids. Perhaps studies in a new field would help. She was very aesthetically inclined. Perhaps an art course?

Three years passed, and the second round came. It was worse this time. Sasha underwent a double mastectomy to fight her deadly heredity. She also had all her reproductive organs removed. She endured treatments that left her aching, gasping, and sleepless. But determined, nonetheless.

She went on to win the second round also. By then, though, she realized that the old Sasha was gone—she had died in the war, so to speak. She tried to find her new self.

Sasha began to tattoo her body all over with rejuvenating messages: *The Healing Hand*, *NO FEAR*, a verdant grapevine, and more. She no longer spoke to people about her disease, because they could no longer hear her; their comments burdened her more than they helped.

Sasha's husband unintentionally added complications to the battle. She watched as he was offered many high-powered positions. Initially, she was horrified that he even considered these labor-intensive jobs, which would take him from the family. Afterward, she wanted him to accept one, hoping that her family's impact on the world (in place of her own) would give her a sense of meaning. Simon similarly wanted these positions but also didn't. So he waited as she waged her war.

Then came the third round. The cancer had spread to bones, organs, and pancreas. She was tired. She was scarred. But she fought on. Sasha entered an experimental drug program.

At the same time, she continued to search for meaning. She deepened her art studies, but in a limited way: "I don't want anything long term. I don't know if I have the time." She produced outstanding work, striving for excellence and creativity as had always been her wont. Sometimes she was able to express her pain, her fears, and her hopes through her art. But she felt this expression sometimes weakened rather than strengthened her. Her interest in art waned.

Sasha then decided to begin participating in medical conferences that discussed the experimental drug she was taking. She was the quintessential speaker; poised, lovely, humorous. Everyone loved her.

Sasha would also speak to new patients, helping them navigate the complexities of the path through their disease. Then, she would return home to fight her own battle.

The experimental drug study continued, losing one participant after another, while Sasha held on for more than two years. An unprecedented success story. Who would have imagined it?

But who knew the price of her success?

She had reinvented herself so many times it was unthinkable. How many more times could she keep doing it? How much helplessness could she tolerate? How much physical, mental, and emotional suffering could she carry? And for what?

Does this story have a happy ending? I don't know. As I write, Sasha's battle continues. It's a "game of thrones" with real blood.

She is now the last survivor in the experimental drug program. Her doctors are excited. But Sasha feels like the proverbial sword of Damocles is swinging just overhead.

At our last meeting, I reminded her, "Your life is also significant because of the drug trial."

The corner of her mouth rose slightly in a tired-looking smirk. "That's not enough," she said. "I need to do something more significant."

"What about the afterlife?" I asked.

"I *don't want* an afterlife," she said through clenched teeth, "I want *this* life!"

I changed tack accordingly. "What about your children? You're significant to them, and through them."

Her eyes wandered down to the worn carpet below us. "I won't even be here to raise them," she said, her voice softly cracking.

We sat in silence for a short time. "You know," I then said quietly, "On that front, you have already won. Psychology claims that the human personality is solidified by the age of eight. Your youngest child is eight."

She smiled a real smile . . . the first one I had seen in a long time.

NOTES TO THE PRACTITIONER

As supporting professionals, we need to align our goal as much as possible with the patient's goal. We must see our patients where they are, stand with them wherever they currently stand, and move with them as they move. This is especially vital in a recurring disease, where the patient's goals can change with each round.

When the patient wants to fight the disease (not always the case; and when it is, it's not necessarily a permanent decision), it is our job to stand with her. Whether it is a battle to participate in an experimental study or to continue treatment, the type of support you give will depend on whether you are a medical or a psychosocial professional. In that capacity, be honest with your patients and/or clients and allow them the right to make informed decisions about their bodies and lives.

"[As a professional,] don't be afraid to suggest or gently broach the subject. For example: "Many of the people I care for in your situation have all sorts of issues that they would like to discuss but are hesitant to do so; is that true for you, too?" Do not be afraid to do this. If the patient doesn't want to talk about something, they will either say, "No, I have no issues," or they will say, "I don't want to talk about this," or they will change the subject. As long as you leave the patient in control, there is little to fear. The chances are that they will be grateful to you for helping them overcome their hesitancy. . . . Don't force anything [and] the patient will lead you where they want, and where they feel safe." (Personal correspondence from Yoram Singer, MD)

Sasha fought her disease because she wanted to live long enough to raise her children. She was far from finished by the time her disease appeared to win in a final way. But she had managed to buy her and her girls at least eight more years of time, and in so doing she passed a pivotal milestone in parenting. Thus, even partial achievement of a goal can be, and should be, acknowledged as a win.

CONCLUSIONS

- *Listen carefully to those in your care; they will help you understand how best to support them. Once you have ascertained what they are asking for, you can make a professional decision. In any case, support them if you can; and if you can't, tell them why without judgment.*
- *The path of the dying patient is not always clear; some want to fight all the time, some want to fight some of the time, and some want to stop fighting. For most, the path changes or wavers frequently. Try to hear the patient at each stage of the battle.*

RECOMMENDED READING

1. "From Fighter to Survivor: 5 Ways Palliative Care Can Help Cancer Patients," July 2019, http://ardenthapc.com/2019/07/24/from-fighter-to-survivor-5-ways-palliative-care-can-help-cancer-patients/ (accessed July 26, 2021).
2. "Dying in Peace and Why Some People Don't," April 2019, https://hospicecarelc.org/dying-in-peace-why-some-people-dont/ (accessed July 26, 2021).

5

cᴎ₂

It Takes a Village

Where Culture Defines Us

Years ago, my colleague Yoram, a palliative physician, told me about a project of his. He drove to the Bedouin* settlements in the southern deserts of Israel, to provide home-hospice services. Ever since I heard about it, I was interested in going with him, to see what this effort looked like.

Such an outreach was complicated. I had only ever seen Bedouin villages from the highway when passing by. They looked like little slums. The houses seemed to be made of corrugated metal, with discarded cars, trucks, and isolated scraps right outside their doors. Goats wandered around, sometimes camels also, and the roads to and from these settlements were bumpy, hole-pocked, axle-breaking traps. Most villages couldn't even be reached without a jeep; Yoram had fundraised the money in order to purchase one for his endeavor.

Finally, I was able to accompany him to these homes.

We two met, and then we were picked up by the four-by-four vehicle with a Bedouin driver. Around 45 minutes later, we arrived at one of the dwellings. The driver had to wait in the jeep, because no men other than family members were allowed into the home. Yoram could go in only because he was a physician.

Once we left the jeep, I realized that under the corrugated metal was a solid concrete building. We knocked, and a woman answered the door in a

* https://www.knesset.gov.il/lexicon/eng/bedouim_eng.htm

Clearing the Path. Lynne Dale Halamish and Eric J. Cassell, Oxford University Press. © Lynne Dale Halamish 2022.
DOI: 10.1093/oso/9780197636879.003.0005

traditional-looking Bedouin gown, all smiles as she greeted the doctor. We entered a salon area, with low couches against the walls and carpets on the floor. In the center of the room was the patient, a woman, lying in a hospital bed. She looked to be in her early 80s (although my Western eyes may have misled me).

There were 10 or 11 other women in the room, of various ages ranging from 5 to 90 years old. Four of them surrounded the patient's bed. Two were massaging her feet and legs with some kind of oil, one was trying to get her to swallow some liquid, and the last was leaning over her, with her ear to the patient's mouth, listening for words that were softly and haltingly spoken in Bedawi Arabic.

Only one of the women knew Hebrew. She spoke to Yoram, loudly complaining that she wanted her mother to be up and about already—and why on earth it was taking so long? Yoram calmly and patiently explained, clearly not for the first time, that her mother would not be recovering from this illness. He asked whether she was sleeping well at night, and if the pain was sufficiently under control.

After a few moments, another woman (the patient's sister, I thought, judging by her age and appearance) approached me with a photo album. She pointed out the patient laughing and dancing at a family celebration only a year earlier, eagerly explaining, in broken Hebrew with pantomime thrown in, "That is what we want!"

A younger woman entered through the hallway with a tray of refreshments: tea, dates, nuts, cashews, and cookies. The younger children's eyes sparkled as they came forward; but following a sharp word from one of the women, they retreated again to their places. "Please," our hostess offered, gesturing to the tray of refreshments.

Yoram and I shared some tea with the women, Yoram quietly speaking words of comfort to them the whole time. After we were done with our repast, the children were allowed to partake.

Yoram then examined his patient, gently touching her and explaining what he was doing so that the Hebrew speaker could translate, while smiling softly at the patient.

I peeked into the hallway and saw many rooms leading off from it. This home was not nearly as small as I had assumed.

Women were coming in and out of the salon, while some sat on the low couches doing needlework. They were all murmuring together, their eyes never leaving the patient or Yoram for long.

After about 45 minutes, Yoram and I said our farewells. He told them when he would return, what he could do to help, and what he could not do. We returned to the jeep and headed for the next home visit.

I asked Yoram, "Were all those women here because you were coming?"

"No," he explained, "they are always with her." He paused. "They are very poor."

"No," I replied thoughtfully. "*We* are very poor. *They* are very rich. In all my years working with the dying, I have never seen so many people care for one dying person like that."

Yoram nodded his head and smiled his gentle smile.

NOTES TO THE PRACTITIONER

We are usually aware, in a general kind of way, that we are "not to judge a book by its cover." However, our visual perceptions tend to color our opinions, particularly in cross-cultural interactions. In our attempts to make a more "orderly" world, we want to classify situations as, for example, "third world" or "primitive," or other labels that frequently carry negative associations and prideful, condescending attitudes.

In multicultural societies, different cultures are often thrown together in settings that are already stressful in themselves: hospitals, courts, police stations, and so on. In these environments, we tend to judge those around us by our own norms.

Whether we intend it or not, this judgment affects the care that we as practitioners provide, in ways that may be unfairly adverse, or unfairly advantageous, to one or more groups. We need to be alert against creating gaps of any kind in the quality of our care.

"It is wise to identify and differentiate between curing and healing. There was no possibility of curing in the story illustrated here. However:

    a. We came to her home.

    b. We stayed with her for 45 minutes.

    c. Yoram touched and examined her, although there was nothing diagnostic to be gained by this examination.

    d. We accepted tea and the food that was offered to us, a sign of respect.

    e. They were grateful that we came, and they were able to make us grateful, too.

All of these, were, in fact, part of a healing process."

(Personal correspondence from Yoram Singer, M.D.)

CONCLUSIONS

- *In combating implicit bias in health and psychological care, we should use the efficient tool of education, and more specifically hands-on education through fieldwork.*

- *In order to avoid disparity in care, it is necessary to first identify and test our own unconscious biases.*
- *Healing can be carried out regardless of the medical situation confronting us.*

RECOMMENDED READING

1. Jillian A. Rose, "The Role of Implicit Bias and Culture in Managing or Navigating Healthcare, Adapted from a Presentation at the SLE Workshop at Hospital for Special Surgery," May 2020, https://www.hss.edu/conditions_role-implicit-bias-culture-managing-navigating-healthcare.asp (accessed July 26, 2021).
2. Zinaria Williams, "Racial Bias in Medicine: A Subconscious Barrier to COVID-19 Equity," January 2021, https://www.usnews.com/news/health-news/articles/2021-01-14/racial-bias-in-medicine-a-barrier-to-covid-health-equity (accessed July 26, 2021).
3. Northwestern Health Unit, "About Health Equity: Equity vs Equality" (n.d.), https://www.healthequitymatters.ca/health-equity/ (accessed July 26, 2021).

6

cVo

Legacy

Choosing What to Leave Behind

"What can I leave to my children?" Susan asked. She was a 67-year-old single mother of four children in their 30s, and this question was posed about 10 days after she was diagnosed with stage-four inoperable cancer.

I answered it with another question. "What would you *like to* leave to them?"

"Well . . ." Susan's eyes wandered as she thought. "I made sure to write a will. I've put their names on my car registration and the deed to my house."

"Very good."

"I've even filled out advance medical directives, so they are not forced to assume responsibility for those decisions . . . I've laid it all out in detail."

"That's good also," I replied.

"So . . . What else can I do?" Susan asked me.

I smiled and said, "You are 67 years old, Susan." I paused and went on. "It looks like your life will not be very much longer than that. What have you learned in your 67 years on this planet?"

"What?" She seemed startled by the question.

"What are some pearls of wisdom, even little ones, that you would like your children to know about? Maybe to emulate? Your priorities. Your values."

"Oh." She thought for a moment, and then seemed to dismiss the idea. "They already know what's important to me. I raised them."

Clearing the Path. Lynne Dale Halamish and Eric J. Cassell, Oxford University Press. © Lynne Dale Halamish 2022.
DOI: 10.1093/oso/9780197636879.003.0006

"Don't be so sure," I cautioned. "You can only know that they know, if you actually write it out clearly."

Susan was still not convinced. "Why would I do that?"

"Your house has value, certainly, and perhaps other possessions as well. But the wisdom you have gathered throughout your life also has value—and in many cases, it's much more valuable than your material possessions."

She pondered for a moment. "I wouldn't know how to do it, though," she finally mumbled.

"Well, I can give you a rough outline if you're interested. Are you?"

"Yes, please." She used her hands to straighten her back and sit up.

"You can begin with the title, 'Legacy.' You should also date it, because you never know if you might want to change it at some point. Subtitle, 'What I would like to leave to my children and their children.' Then you list values and important lessons learned from your birth until now. Keep in mind that some of these values may change between now and the day of your death. Then end it with, 'This is my Legacy to you, my children, grandchildren, and future generations. Do with it what you will. Take it and apply it, or throw it away.'"

I continued, "The main thing is to write down things that are important to you, or lessons you have learned in the course of your life. You can write it as one long story or divide it with titles; make the style formal or informal. It can include things you have done, right or wrong, as well as things not done that you understand that you should have done."

Then I named a few examples of what she could include in such a legacy.

PARENTHOOD

My four children are amazing, wise in many ways, foolish in some. I have had the privilege of seeing three of them become spouses and parents. Thoughtful, contemplative, attentive parents who listen to their children, who guide them. Who bless them.

YOUR NAME

Guard your reputation. Do not besmirch yourself. It is almost impossible to clean off any mud you allow to settle on your name. Do not lie for anything less than hiding innocent people from murderers. Do not ally yourselves with immoral people. This will taint your name.

"And you can go on from there," I concluded, "writing about things that you feel are important for them to know, when you are no longer there to guide them."

Susan was silent for a moment. "I would like to talk to them about responsibility," she added thoughtfully. "Maybe something like . . .

"'Take responsibility for your life, whatever your circumstances are. It doesn't matter what the situation is, you can take responsibility and improve it. Or you can blame the world, the boss, the country, and sit impotently by. But that's a waste of energy and personal resources. I have witnessed the incredible bravery of people who have less than nothing, and have done so much with it. I have witnessed others who have an abundance of everything, and are so poor in their own eyes, so victimized, that they are completely neutralized.' How does that sound?"

"Great!" I replied sincerely. Susan may have been surprised by the idea of a legacy, but I saw her enthusiasm build as we spoke.

"Oh, I know another one," she added suddenly. "'In light of this surprise cancer I got, I would also like to say: Use the fancy dishes TODAY!'" She smiled and nodded.

"Very good and true," I responded.

She continued with the same thought. "'Today is all you have. Whether or not you have tomorrow, no one knows. If you have lovely dishes that you are 'saving for a special occasion,' use them today.'"

When we met again a month later, Susan's health had clearly deteriorated. However, she came to our meeting with a notebook. Proudly she showed me copies of her legacy, in four plastic-covered sheets, that she had made for her children.

NOTES TO THE PRACTITIONER

The question of significance is a huge part of who we are as humans. The need to make important or noteworthy contributions which have consequences, relevance, valuable content, and/or historic merit doesn't cease to be important to us when we are ill or facing death. Many times (though *not* always), the need becomes even more critical as death approaches.

When your patients or counselees ask what they can leave behind, a legacy of personal values is often a good suggestion. Alternately, depending on how much time is available, they might want to write their own history, which of course is also their family's history.

In my experience, this can be both a rewarding and daunting task. Those who are intimidated by the idea can accomplish it by working with a ghostwriter, which has its own benefits. Ghostwriters can occupy a great deal of the patient's idle time with interviews, distracting from fears, and sometimes even from pain. They come up with a reasonable finished product that one can leave behind for the family.

I have also accompanied people who wanted to leave a video eulogy that can be viewed during the mourning period.

Whatever its form, the specific message can be anything significant to the dying person. The search for it, and the expression of it, is part of this perhaps final journey. It can be a personal vision statement, or a family vision that connects several generations. It can contain values combined with forecasts, and/or ideals with subjective intrinsic value, whether or not they have been accomplished during the subject's life. All of these options carry value both to the patient and possibly also to the family.

CONCLUSIONS

- *A quest for significance, and the task of expressing it, can frequently help patients experience a meaningful "last journey" before their death.*
- *Such a legacy can also become a gift for other family members when one is facing death.*

RECOMMENDED READING

1. Ana Cocarla, "Finding Meaning and Purpose in Old Age," *Emoha Elder Care*, May 2020, https://emoha.com/blogs/give-back/finding-meaning-and-purpose-old-age (accessed July 26, 2021).
2. Dawn Franks, "How to Write a Legacy Statement—The Most Important Gift You Will Leave Behind," *Your Philanthropy*, March 2018, https://your-philanthr opy.com/write-Legacy-statement/ (accessed July 26, 2021).

7

⌘

Last Respects

Communication with Patient and Family

I was giving a seminar to the nursing and support staff in a primarily geriatric and palliative care hospital. My topic was communication with
dying patients.

Before I had gotten very far, one of the nurses protested, "That's all very
well, but we don't have time to do this with the patients."

Seeing signs of strong emotion, I replied, "Talk to me."

She began to elaborate, backed by murmurs of agreement from those
surrounding her.

"Just this week we had a terrible situation. A young mother of three who
was dying. It was horrible. Her whole extended family was gathered around
her, except for the children. They were all screaming and wailing and yelling
at the staff and crying. So was she. She was here for an entire week, and we
couldn't get her pain under control. She died an awful death, because we
just couldn't help her."

All the staff members around her were nodding in agreement. Some
were even holding their heads in their hands or covering their eyes, reliving
the pain. It was clear they had all been through a traumatic event.

I was silent for a moment and then asked, "Did anyone else who was
young die here this week?"

She replied thoughtfully, "Well, yes. . . . There was another young woman
with three young children. The whole family was present there also . . . including her children. They were all very quiet and soft-spoken; we kept

Clearing the Path. Lynne Dale Halamish and Eric J. Cassell, Oxford University Press. © Lynne Dale Halamish 2022.
DOI: 10.1093/oso/9780197636879.003.0007

asking if they needed anything, and they kept refusing politely. The woman died peacefully, and the family thanked us and brought us chocolates. She was here for only three days."

Again, the staff members were nodding their heads along with the story; only now they were smiling at the memory of this young woman's peaceful end. A woman the same age as some of the nurses sitting in the room.

"Was her name Helen?" I asked.

Startled, the nurse replied, "Yes, it was! How did you know?"

"She was a client of mine," I replied.

"But," she said, "you must have had loads of time working with her, probably months."

"No, I had one 90-minute meeting with her," I replied. "And before that, I met just three times with her husband."

"Okay," the nurse conceded. "But we don't even have 90 minutes to spare for each of our terminal patients! How could we possibly have any meaningful, game-changing communication with them?"

"It doesn't have to be in one sitting. You can have several 10-minute sessions."

I let the idea float in the silence that now filled the room. I continued with practical tools:

"When you admit a new patient, ask them what they know about their reasons for coming here. You want to know if they know they are terminally ill. Ask them if they have someone to help them emotionally during this difficult time. You have a social worker on your staff, and she can be offered as an option. If she feels unequal to the task, she can get additional training."

"You can also choose to refer patients to a hospice social worker, or a palliative professional counselor, who can meet with the patient's spouse or primary caregiver. They can meet with the whole family if needed."

A wave of relief and surprise passed over the faces in the room. Could these dedicated caregivers delegate some of the emotional burden of the families of their patients to outside resources?

I smiled and continued, "Your part in the communication is mostly about giving dying patients and their family someone to speak to, openly, about the illness. You are someone who can tell them about its usual course, which symptoms may appear, and what to expect at the end. This helps the family gain a sense of control, so that they can plan how to meet the approaching death. On the emotional side, it helps the dying person to start the separation process from their children, from their spouse, and from their own body."

"The first time you're involved in this kind of communication, it will be difficult. But once you witness the benefits for the family, for the patient—for you and everyone else around them—it will become not only doable, but easier. At the end of the day, this conversation takes less time and effort than trying to handle the panic surrounding a lonely, uninformed, unsupported patient. As you already saw, just because family is around doesn't mean the patient has support."

I returned to the incident they had shared with me, focusing on their helplessness to relieve the dying patient's pain.

"Sometimes, pain is intractable because it's exacerbated by fear. In those cases, it can help to use anti-anxiety and anti-depression medications along with the pain-control meds. Even more helpful is just taking a few minutes to listen to the patient. Be open and honest, be respectful, and allow silence to reign where it's appropriate."

I continued: "That may not sound like much, but from my experience it really does make a difference—not only for the patient and family, but for the staff or anyone who is trying to help. If the dying person can express their fear, and know that they have been 'heard,' the inner tension may subside enough to allow the painkillers to do their work."

NOTES TO THE PRACTITIONER

In both of the cases mentioned here, the time period between admission and death was relatively short. The intervention recommended was also short term.

While scarcity of time is a dominant factor for medical caregivers, it's even a more pressing issue for the dying patient. The competing demands on time can be particularly distressing for hospital staff, who are often short-handed. However, all too frequently more time is spent trying to navigate around a distressed, panicky family than the time it would take to assist them by listening.

The length of time is not critical; in fact, end-of-life (EOL) patients often don't have the strength for a long-winded intervention. Ten-minute conversations, with the promise to return in a short time for another 10-minute talk, can be equally effective. The segmentation also helps the patient focus on specific issues each time.

Whether the dying person is at home or in hospital, it's helpful to find outside mental health professionals who can assist the families and close friends of the patient. Although we should pay attention to the family as well, our main focus as the EOL counselor must be on the patient.

If the institutional support staff—the social worker, psychologist, or spiritual counselor —feels inadequate to assist dying patients and their family in preparing for death, the wise manager will make sure that key personnel receive the necessary additional training, as it will benefit the entire staff.

In many cases involving anxiety and fear, a delay in using pharmacological assistance to reduce the anxiety can exacerbate the pain level, thereby increasing the panic. Early intervention is usually extremely effective.

CONCLUSIONS

- *It is worthwhile to assess, upon admission, the EOL patient's awareness of their condition, and the support structure around them, in order to supplement that support where needed.*
- *Sometimes families need external psychological support to deal with their impending loss.*
- *If you don't have the time for a lengthy meeting with the patient, a few short talks can be just as effective and perhaps even more so.*
- *Once the patients feel "heard," they tend to relax as the communication improves; this in turn can help alleviate both emotional anxiety and physical pain.*

RECOMMENDED READING

1. I. Timmers, A. L. Kaas, C. W. E. M. Quaedflieg, et al., "Fear of Pain and Cortisol Reactivity Predict the Strength of Stress-Induced Hypoalgesia," *European Journal of Pain* 22(7) (August 19, 2018): 1291–1303, https://www.ncbi.nlm.nih.gov/pmc/articles/PMC6055649/, doi:10.1002/ejp.1217 (accessed July 27, 2021).
2. Indrany Datta-Barua and Joshua Hauser, "Four Communication Skills from Psychiatry Useful in Palliative Care and How to Teach Them," *AMA Journal of Ethics* (August 2018), https://journalofethics.ama-assn.org/article/four-communication-skills-psychiatry-useful-palliative-care-and-how-teach-them/2018-08 (accessed July 27, 2021).

II

Preparing Children for a Death

8

❧

Plan B

Using Teachable Moments with Children

Mercy was just 7 years old. Her mother was dying from stage-four cancer.

I was meeting with Henry, her father. We had been talking about helping him to find a way to talk to Mercy about her mother's imminent death, in order to prepare her.

"How can I tell her? She is too young."

"Henry," I replied, "you have two advantages. You have Mercy's trust as her father, and you have time on your side. Time to say goodbye to your wife, and to help your child say goodbye to her mother. Don't waste it. You are already paying the price of an extended illness. Take the benefit, too. Pay attention to Mercy and watch for a teachable moment. It will come."

Three days later, Mercy came home from school and said to her father, "I can't wait till Mom comes home from the hospital again! I miss her . . . And you know what? If she *doesn't* die, if she *beats* the cancer, you know what we'll do? We'll throw a big party for her! We will invite everyone. We'll have lots of food and a really great time!"

This was the first time the word "die" had been mentioned. And it came out of the 7-year-old's mouth.

Her father looked at her for a moment. "Mercy, you know what?"

"What, Dad?"

He took a few steps towards Mercy and sat beside her on the couch before answering. "If she beats the cancer, that's exactly what we will do.

Clearing the Path. Lynne Dale Halamish and Eric J. Cassell, Oxford University Press. © Lynne Dale Halamish 2022.
DOI: 10.1093/oso/9780197636879.003.0008

But if she doesn't beat the cancer, and she dies, do you know what we will do then?"

"What?"

"We will have a funeral. And after that, we will have Shiva.* Do you know what happens during Shiva?"

"What?"

"We will be at home for 7 days, and many people will come to visit us. We will look at pictures of Mom together, and we will tell people about her, and they will tell us about her, too. There will also be food. It will be hard. And sad. But we will be together."

"Ok, Dad, that's exactly what we'll do."

NOTES TO THE PRACTITIONER

When dealing with young children, death in the family seems an impossible subject to raise, even when it is imminent. But death from illness is also an opportunity; the intervening time can be used for communication that will prepare the children and the patient for the coming separation. If we don't use this opportunity, the child will pay a double price: dealing with their anxiety for the sick family member, *and* dealing with the shock of a sudden, unexpected death.

People of all ages usually manage grief better with some preparation where possible. Children can cope, many times even better than the adults around them, with difficult information. Being included in the grieving group, including anticipatory grief, is preferable to being left to cope alone; and children are no different in that respect.

If the family is directed to pay close attention to the children, they will usually discover that the children are more aware of the situation than they thought. The key is listening carefully, asking about dreams, thoughts, drawings, or casual comments made by the child. Also asking open questions like "Why is Mom in the hospital?" and other concrete subjects (see Chapters 9, 10, and 13) can help adults assess what the children know, and any misconceptions they might be harboring about what is going on.

---

* *Shiva*, meaning "seven" in Hebrew, is the Jewish custom in which family members of the deceased gather for 7 days after the burial and mourn their loss. This is conducted in an informal open-house atmosphere, which encourages friends and neighbors to drop in, bring food, and share their memories of the deceased to comfort the mourners.

CONCLUSIONS

- *Use teachable moments to prepare children for an impending death.*
- *Presenting a concrete plan of action is important in giving children ways to cope. So is an alternate plan, if the future is uncertain.*

RECOMMENDED READING

1. Anna C. Muriel, "Preparing Children and Adolescents for the Loss of a Loved One," May 2021, *UpToDate*, https://www.uptodate.com/contents/preparing-children-and-adolescents-for-the-loss-of-a-loved-one (accessed July 27, 2021).
2. "How to Prepare a Child for the Death of a Parent by Cancer," *Winston's Wish Advice*, February 4, 2019, https://www.winstonswish.org/prepare-death-by-cancer/ (accessed July 27, 2021).

9

Denial

Blessing the Children Before You Go

Jonathan called me with a problem: the 34-year-old man's wife was dying and refused to face it, talk about it, or prepare for it. He said, "Goldie doesn't even know she is dying. Could you help us, so that she can at least say goodbye to our three children [aged 3, 5, and 7]?"

In my experience, dying people know that they are dying, whether they're 90 years old or 5. In fact, I personally have never met a person who was dying and did not know it.

Goldie was a 32-year-old woman with advanced cancer. When I met her, she weighed 30 kg (66 lb) and had a catheter and a nose tube.

When I arrived at their home, I asked to speak to her alone.

Why? Generally speaking, family members in this kind of situation try to "protect" one another, which leads to a tendency to hide their fears or pain from each other. But the dying person needs to be able to talk about the approaching death.

As Goldie began to talk, it quickly became apparent that she was indeed dying, and that she was well aware of it.

I gave her "center stage," allowing her to speak unhindered, only asking questions now and then in a low voice for minimal interruption.

At one point she asked me, "How will I die?"

It is important (especially for medical personnel) to recognize that most people have never witnessed a real death and have no idea what to expect. Where does the average person get their impressions about death?

Clearing the Path. Lynne Dale Halamish and Eric J. Cassell, Oxford University Press. © Lynne Dale Halamish 2022.
DOI: 10.1093/oso/9780197636879.003.0009

Sensationalized scenes from movies, Internet, or television, which some-times include screams, blood everywhere, horror stories, and fear of the unknown. This frequently causes frank disbelief in family members when they witness the death of their loved one occurring quietly and calmly, without extra drama.

Giving information to the families who are facing death, concerning what to expect, usually provides an anchor for them and is greatly appreciated.

Given Goldie's medical condition, I described a likely scenario of her death.

Goldie wept a bit, and said, "I am so relieved. I was very afraid it would be horrific."

"Goldie, what is hardest for you right now?" I asked after a pause.

Her answer revealed her own view of the problem her husband had described. "I can't stand how Jonathan always wants to talk about my impending death."

When a couple is dealing with the torrent of emotions caused by approaching death, it is extremely rare to find both processing this at the same pace or in the same manner One partner usually wants to talk, while the other would prefer not to. What should the compromise be in this case? When they contradict each other strongly enough to make compromise dif-ficult, whose wishes should be respected?

"Would you like me to talk to him, Goldie?"

She immediately agreed and called her husband in to sit with us; and as he sat down, I said:

"Jonathan, Goldie has a terrible disease. You know this, and so does she."

Clarification in simple language is a big part of effective communication. We were all quiet for a moment. Then I continued.

"She probably won't survive this disease. You know this, and so does she."

This clarification was important to state with both of them present. Its purpose was to break down barriers to mutual understanding. It wasn't the time to communicate about the issues creating tension between them, which Goldie didn't want to do at this point. We needed to clarify and re-move the friction point which she had chosen as "the hardest right now" for her.

And in this case, it could be done fairly easily. Jonathan wouldn't need to insist that Goldie admit that she is dying if he could see that she already knows it.

I paused, and then went on. "It's her body and her fight. So, Goldie decides when, where, what, and to whom she wants to talk about it; be-cause it is her life and her loss."

I paused again. What I had just said was true. However, it is also important for each listener to "see" their partner, to recognize and legitimatize what he or she is experiencing.

I turned to Jonathan. "It's clear that you have many losses here also. You have lost your healthy wife, your secure future, and the secure future of your children. But her losses are even bigger and harder, so she decides when and how she can talk about it."

I continued: "So . . . If you need to talk to someone when Goldie doesn't want to talk, you can talk to me. Or to anyone else that you would like to. Just not Goldie."

Goldie seemed quite relieved as Jonathan agreed to this arrangement. We were now free to address the other concern which Jonathan had mentioned to me: the three young children who were about to lose their mother.

I turned to her. "You know, a parent is a mirror for her child. Once the parent is gone, the mirror doesn't exist anymore. Would you like to be that mirror and bless your children* before you go?"

Goldie was delighted with the idea. She was happy to have a significant project that she could actually do. And she was relieved at still having some way to protect her children, both by giving them their "mirror" of how she saw them and to help them remember her.

Since she was still able to write, she worked out a plan with me to write to each child individually. Each blessing would begin with the story of that child's life from their mother's perspective. How did Goldie feel when she first found out she was pregnant with him or her? How were the pregnancy and the birth? How was a name decided on, and what is the significance of the name? I asked her to choose memories she wanted to preserve in writing, of interactions with the child and what she sees as his or her strengths . . . as well as vulnerable points that will need watching as they grow. She would end each blessing with a meaningful declaration of her love, and that she never intended to leave them so soon.

Afterwards, her original handwritten letters could be taken to a calligrapher, or her original handwriting could be reproduced on good paper in two copies, one for Jonathan to save and one for the children to receive when she said goodbye to them. If Goldie had been unwilling or unable to write, she could have made a video or audio recording to be transcribed (or kept in electronic form).

---

* For more details, see Chapters 6 (Legacy) and/or 17 (Blessing and Cursing).

It was very hard for Goldie to say goodbye to her children. This strategy of reframing the goodbye into a blessing essentially helped her to handle this separation in a healthy way for all concerned.

Goldie wrote out her blessings and spoke to each of her children. We met twice more before her situation deteriorated and she had to be hospitalized. She died peacefully there.

NOTES TO THE PRACTITIONER

When meeting a patient or a client, especially one who has not initiated the meeting, it is important to hear their story, and not depend on the story someone else has told you about them. During that narrative, any need for clarification should be expressed in a low, quiet question; this usually does not interrupt the flow of the narrative the way a question in a regular tone does.

To the individual who is facing death, most of their control has been taken away over many aspects of their life. Therefore, it is important to give them control over anything that they can still manage, in order to fight feelings of helplessness engendered by the reality of their situation.

"There is usually an inherent need for the dying patient to be able to talk about imminent death. Many people who do not or cannot talk about this will experience extreme loneliness." (Personal correspondence from Yoram Singer, MD)

When a conflict of interests arises between the needs of the patient and the needs of a family member, it is possible to look for a creative way to assist the family member. I do, however, usually emphasize the rights of the dying person.

Even while moving towards death, a meaningful task like the blessings described in this case may be of great comfort to a dying parent, or a dying child.

CONCLUSIONS

- *People who are dying are usually aware of it.*
- *Dying patients should be allowed to speak on the subject of impending death as they choose, deciding when, where, in how much detail, and with whom to speak; or to refrain from speaking, if that is their desire.*

• *Parents who are dying should be given the tools to bless their children and to share their history with the child through the eyes of the parent.*

RECOMMENDED READING

1.   Dana Sparks, "Science Saturday: Hospice Research to Understand the Process of Dying and End-of-Life Care," *Mayo Clinic News Network* (September 7, 2019), https://newsnetwork.mayoclinic.org/discussion/science-saturday-hospice-research-to-understand-process-of-dying-and-end-of-life-care/ (accessed July 27, 2021).
2.   Meredith Begley, "Hard Conversations: How to Talk to Your Care Team and Loved Ones about Dying," *Memorial Sloan Kettering Cancer Center* (June 20, 2019), https://www.mskcc.org/news/hard-conversations-how-talk-your-care-team-and-loved-ones-about-dying (accessed July 27, 2021).

10

ᬣᬥ

Carpet Talk

Talking to Small Children about
a Dying Classmate

Sandy, a 4-year-old boy, had stage-four cancer. His kindergarten teacher, Susan, called me to schedule a meeting.

"I am worried," she explained at our meeting. "The other kids are talking about Sandy, saying all kinds of strange things."

"What do you do when they talk about him?" I asked her.

"I just listen."

"When the kids talk about other things, do you just listen or do you join in?"

She thought for a moment. "I usually join in."

"Why is this subject different?"

She paused, searching for an honest answer. "I'm afraid."

"What are you afraid of?" I persisted.

"It might hurt the children to talk about it."

"But you said they are already talking about it."

"Yes. . . . They are."

I remained silent for a moment and then asked her: "What else about this frightens you?"

"What if they ask me a question that I can't answer?"

"What do you do when they ask you other questions that you can't answer?"

Clearing the Path. Lynne Dale Halamish and Eric J. Cassell, Oxford University Press. © Lynne Dale Halamish 2022.
DOI: 10.1093/oso/9780197636879.003.0010

"I usually ask, 'What do you think?' to get their answers. Then I say, 'So, some people think this and others think that.' Or, sometimes I say, 'I'll find out the answer and I'll tell you about it later.'"

When children ask a question, it is wise to ask them the same question back—using the same words if possible—and then listen to their answer before providing them with your own. The first part ensures that we understand what their question is, while the second part reveals whether they are laboring under any misconceptions. Giving our answer without doing this is like shooting in the dark: We have no idea where to aim to provide them with the information they need.

I turned to Susan. "You're an educator of these children. They need to understand that they can talk about this with you, and that you are willing both to listen to what they have to say about it, and to talk about it yourself."

Susan thought for a moment and then looked down. "I *can't* talk to them about it. I don't know how . . ."

I replied, "Okay. It's okay, really. Let's find a time when I can come and meet the children."

It is hard to break the taboos surrounding death just on the strength of a mental recognition that this should be part of an educator's job. It is easier if the teacher sees the theory in action. Susan needed to observe that children are not hurt by talking about death and illness, but rather they benefit from it.

"In two days," I said, "I will come to the kindergarten. Please arrange for the children to sit on a carpet on the floor with me. All kindergarten staff must be present to hear what is said, and to see and hear the children's responses. Your quiet participation is a way of confirming to them that you agree with what I am saying, so that everyone is on the same page. The other staff members will also see that talking about this subject does not harm the children, but rather helps them. Then, later, if the children have additional questions, you will all be able to answer in accordance with what you have heard in the meeting."

Two days later, I entered the children's library, a carpeted room with a large space in the middle. The 16 children were herded in by the teacher and her two assistants, who instructed the youngsters to sit with me in a circle on the carpet. They were in high spirits as they jostled for their places around the circle; they could tell something new was happening.

I sat on the floor with them, rather than on a chair, to remain physically on the same level with them. This is generally a good way to help children to feel comfortable with an adult and with what would be said.

"Hi, kids," I began with a smile.

They said, "Hi" back, some attentive, some still jostling with their neighbors.

"So, how are you today?"

Various answers are heard around the circle: "Good," "Fine," and so on.

The most effective way to communicate with children (and probably with adults, too) is through questions rather than statements. Questions make the session interactive rather than passive; that in turn opens a window into what they are thinking or feeling.

"So, where is Sandy?" I began.

A couple of the children volunteered an answer: "Sandy is sick, he can't come today."

"Does anybody know what the name of Sandy's sickness is?"

"Cancer!" was shouted out from various directions around the circle.

"What is cancer?" I asked.

"It's a sickness!"

"My Grandpa has it!" called out one child.

"My uncle died from it!" added another.

"How do you get it?" I asked.

A momentary silence fell over the room. The kids looked around and started comparing their thoughts with one another.

"Is cancer contagious?" I asked.

Some of the children said yes, and others said no. "What does 'contagious' mean?" one asked.

Another child answered, "It means that one person can get sick from another person."

"That's right," I said. "How does that happen?"

"When the sick person sneezes or coughs," replied one of the kids.

"So, is cancer contagious?" I repeated. Once again, some of the children said yes, and others said no.

Once the room quieted down again, I said. "No. Cancer is not contagious." I paused and then asked, "What kind of sickness *is* contagious?"

"Corona?" asked one child.

"Yes. Colds, and the sniffles, and coronavirus. . . ." I answered. "But cancer is not."

I waited as they processed and compared these familiar examples with Sandy's illness.

"What that means is, you can visit Sandy and you won't get cancer from that. You can play with Sandy, and you won't get cancer from that." I addressed the child who had shared that his grandfather had cancer: "You can hug your grandpa, and you won't get cancer from that either."

I looked around and continued, "You can even eat from the same spoon and not get cancer from it. You can even—*YUCK YUCK YUCK*—brush your teeth with Sandy's toothbrush! And you won't get cancer even from that!"

Gagging sounds, "Yuck," and "Ewww" came from the children, accompanied by the occasional giggle.

The goal here was to prevent the isolation of the ill child. It was also an opportunity to provide accurate and relevant knowledge for other encounters with cancer patients.

"So," I asked, "How do people get cancer?"

"Maybe they are bad people?" said one girl.

"Is Sandy a bad person?" I asked.

"No." They answered without hesitation.

"Is this boy's grandpa a bad person?" I asked.

Again, a firm "no" came from various places in the circle. Another added as proof: "He came to the kindergarten to read us a story once!" The grandchild smiled proudly.

"No, you are right," I agreed with them. "People don't get cancer because they're bad."

"Cigarettes," someone volunteered.

"Well, cigarettes cause cancer sometimes, but Sandy doesn't smoke cigarettes . . . does he?"

"No, no, no—he's too little to smoke."

"Sandy didn't do anything to get cancer. We don't know why he has it; he just does. We don't always have all the answers."

Here, I was emphasizing the lack of guilt on the part of the patient. Believing that someone with a fatal illness must have somehow caused it may offer the temporary relief of "having an answer," but it essentially tells the victim: "Not only are you dying, but you deserve it for your behavior."

"So, what happens when someone has cancer?" I asked.

A voice piped up with a practical answer typical for this age group: "He doesn't come to kindergarten."

Another child challenged that with "But sometimes he does, when he's feeling better."

As I waited and listened, the little girl sitting to my right picked up my hand and began playing with my fingers. The boy on my left leaned his head on my upper arm. I stroked his head with my free hand for a moment, while the observations about Sandy kept coming at a random pace.

"He's always tired."

"He has no hair," said someone. The others started to giggle.

"Why doesn't he have hair?" I asked.

"Because he is sick," answered someone.

"No, it's because of the medicine. If he doesn't have any hair, that means the medicine is working. So, it's actually a good sign." I paused for a moment to let that truth sink in, and then carried on: "Anyway, if he gets better, his hair will grow back."

"If . . ." This was the first time that the possibility had been raised.

"*Will* he get better?" I asked.

The kids started asking each other, "Will he get better?" A few of them were distracted and started shoving each other, and the teacher had to intervene.

"Well, the doctors are trying to make him better. We hope he will," I said. I could feel tension from the kindergarten staff as we neared the borders of that taboo subject. The other "if."

"But he *will* get better, won't he?" asked the girl on my right.

I turned to her: "We hope so. Maybe." I waited a few seconds and then asked: "What will happen if he *doesn't* get better?"

"He won't come back to kindergarten?"

"Yes, that's true. If he doesn't get better, he won't come back to kindergarten." After another pause, I asked, "What else won't he do if he doesn't get better?"

"He won't play."

"My uncle died from it," repeated one of the children. "Could Sandy die?"

There—the dreaded word was uttered—and by one of the children. The staff collectively held their breath, waiting to see how I was going to respond to this.

"People do die from cancer sometimes," I replied after a few seconds.

Someone in the circle demanded a more specific answer. "Will *he* die?"

"He *could*. We hope not, but we don't know for sure," I said.

Do not miss the opportunity of letting children try to answer their own questions. By the same token, do not try to avoid a difficult truth. If your answer to their query is dishonest or too vague, the children will know it on some level. Even small children sense when they cannot speak to us about a certain subject or cannot trust us to tell them the truth.

The kindergarten kids were now becoming restless; their concentration skills had reached their limits. But we had accomplished our goal.

Children have a short attention span, particularly in a group. We don't want to strain that capacity. Nor do we need to. Once the kids know who they can turn to on this subject, they will be less reluctant to bring it up again, whether in the group or individually.

"Who wants to draw a picture for Sandy to cheer him up?" Susan asked.

A chorus of "I do," and "Me, me!" answered her as the kids leaped up and charged at the table with the art materials.

Susan had thought that everything she knew about communicating with small children was suddenly invalidated when it came to talking about terminal cancer. But in reality, all of the standard teaching tools and relating skills that she had honed for years in her work were still just as relevant as ever, if not more so.

There is no reason to leave children alone with their thoughts about sickness and death, which can include both real and imagined fears. Educators have an excellent opportunity to correct misconceptions even among young children—but only after the wrong ideas are identified and replaced with accurate information appropriate for their age.

NOTES TO THE PRACTITIONER

In this case, I emphasize the importance of getting the child's answer to every question of substance, before we give our own. If we provide an answer first, and only then ask children for their answers, we usually receive a version of our own answer. It is more valuable to discover what the child really thinks about the relevant illness, its causes and consequences, in order to discover any misconceptions that need to be cleared up.

When working with someone close to a case of terminal illness or death, there are many societal taboos that need to be overcome. Among them is the notion that children should be "protected" from the truth of an impending death. When the inevitable truth emerges, the lie spoken in misguided kindness will have destroyed the child's trust in the speaker, precisely at the time when it is most needed.

Because professionals themselves are also vulnerable to these taboos, it is often more efficient to demonstrate how to communicate on this subject, rather than to simply direct the professional or the parent.

The first time a counselor is communicating with children about death or impending death, it is valuable to be a silent witness to such a demonstration by a more experienced colleague. The second time, the experienced colleague should participate silently in the meeting while the counselor manages the conversation, and later give pointed, constructive feedback on how the encounter went. Like anything else, this kind of communication needs to be practiced in order to improve.

After an in-class experience such as the one described here, the children should be sent home with a letter informing their parents about the discussion and what transpired in it. Besides keeping the parents informed, it may help them to overcome their own taboos in family discussions about critical illness and death.

CONCLUSIONS

- *Questions provoke significantly more conversation and thoughtfulness than statements do. Questions in response to questions help clarify the original intent.*
- *Lying to children is not a kindness. It is a breach of trust, and it has consequences.*
- *Keep parents informed of discussions conducted with their children about death and dying.*
- *Where possible, try to demonstrate communication techniques, rather than merely explaining them.*
- *The contagiousness of a disease should be made clear to children, in order to prevent distance and isolation where it is unnecessary.*
- *Causes for an illness should be clarified, to avoid condemnation of the patient.*

RECOMMENDED READING

1. Andrea Warnick, "When to Tell the Children: Preparing Children for the Death of Someone Close to Them," *Canadian Virtual Hospice* (May 2019), https://www.virtualhospice.ca/en_US/Main+Site+Navigation/Home/Topics/Topics/Communication/When+to+Tell+the+Children_+Preparing+Children+for+the+Death+of+Someone+Close+to+Them.aspx (accessed July 27, 2021).
2. The Children's Oncology Group, "School Support: Talking with Your Classroom about Cancer," https://www.childrensoncologygroup.org/index.php/school-support (accessed July 27, 2021).

11

꧁

Last Lullaby

Saying Goodbye to Young Children

Marina and Alex, a young couple in their late 30s, called me from the hospital.

Marina was hospitalized for the umpteenth time; this time would be her last.

We had been meeting since shortly after the onset of her disease. More recently, we met several times to work on helping her to say goodbye in general, and particularly to her three small children, all under 10 years old.

Marina began what would be our last conversation.

"I was writing letters to the children, but in the last few days, my body... so weak... has kept me from writing anymore." She sighed. "What do I do with my kids? What do I say? How do I say it? Should I say anything?"

I answered her with practical advice. "I strongly recommend that Alex record you on his cellphone. That way, you can tell the children all the things you are too weak to write. Someone can transcribe it later. This is important. Do it today; don't wait."

There was silence on the other side of the line. All I could hear were Marina's raspy breathing and the faint and steady beeping of the medical monitor in the background. I went on.

"I understand it's difficult for you to say goodbye to your children, because you want to protect them. But preparing them *is* protecting them. If you don't do it, this opportunity for an intimate, significant goodbye will

Clearing the Path. Lynne Dale Halamish and Eric J. Cassell, Oxford University Press. © Lynne Dale Halamish 2022.
DOI: 10.1093/oso/9780197636879.003.0011

be experienced by your children as a sudden unexpected death, with no communication at all."

Marina cleared her throat. "Tell me again, what should I say?"

"Ask your children for forgiveness. Tell them that it's not your desire or intention to leave them. Tell them that you understand that it will hurt them, and you are deeply sorry for that. For example, you can say: 'I don't want to leave. I want to be with you, but my body will not allow me to. I would like to stay with you. You are dear and important to me.'"

"Then say: 'I forgive you for every mistake you ever made. For every time I was irritated or angry with you. For everything you didn't do that needed to be done. I forgive you.'"

I explained, "Children are usually the center of their own world. As a result, they often believe things happen because of their own thoughts, wishes, words, or actions. It's important to explicitly tell your children that there is nothing they did to cause your illness or death, and there was nothing they could have done to prevent it. This is one reason why this talk with your children is so significant. They need for you to absolve them from any unwarranted guilt or at least to reduce it, and to tell them who they are in your eyes.

"Tell them that you love them, and what you love about them. Thank them for what they have been to you. They don't need to be big things, but everything you say needs to be true."

I continued: "After you have said these things to them, together or separately, it will be time to say goodbye. You are very tired already. You can say, 'I love you. In some ways, I will always be with you, like when you see me in your face or in your personality. Half of who you are comes from me, and this you will carry with you throughout your life. I am grateful to have been your mother. Goodbye, my child.'"

"Say goodbye to each one of them. Don't leave anyone out."

Marina succeeded in this final task. Her husband reported that although the children wept, they were comforted by her words and hugs.

NOTES TO THE PRACTITIONER

A terminal illness puts you "on the clock." Whatever needs to be done should be done "now." Whatever time is left after that can be used at will.

When it comes to communication, sooner is better. The inability to communicate can occur well before the actual death. This can be caused by the advancement of the disease, the harshness of the treatments, drug-related reactions, exhaustion, pain, and even fear. With a life-threatening illness, we are racing against time.

Moreover, "safe" is better than "sorry." If something significant is said which turns out to be unnecessary, nothing has been lost. For example, suppose the patient goes into an extended remission of the disease. In that case, nothing negative will occur from the patient having spoken honestly to their family and expressed their love. On the contrary, the communication between family members or loved ones is usually improved.

When someone is facing their illness, the listener should be accompanying them. When they deny the illness, the listener should still be with them, not fighting them. Why? There are really only two human conditions: People are either alive or dead. And when alive, they needn't spend all their time thinking about death, even if it is impending. There are choices to be made surrounding the end of life. But it's natural for them to then return to life or any part of life that remains to them.

When establishing a "new normal," it is essential for the family's children to be as involved as possible—not in the fine details of the illness, but in the emotional side of the experience, so they will not have to walk the path of grief completely alone. Where possible, the children should make visits to the hospital. When this is not possible (as was the case during the COVID-19 pandemic), the tools of Internet video or phone conversations can also help children feel embraced by their families.

Expect, and inform the family to expect, regressive behavior in the children. It can be exemplified in bedwetting, clinginess, or other childish behaviors. This is not a time for discipline, but rather for support, caring, and warmth.

CONCLUSIONS

- *Keep the children involved with their sick family members, arranging communication wherever possible, by whatever means available.*
- *Arrange for significant communication with the ill person as early as possible.*
- *Due to young children's tendency to take responsibility for things that happen around them, they need to be explicitly absolved of guilt surrounding a family member's illness and/or death.*
- *Expect temporary developmental or emotional regression in children in the shadow of serious illness, death, or trauma.*

RECOMMENDED READING

1. Andrea Warnick, "Children at the Bedside of a Dying Family Member or Friend," *Canadian Virtual Hospice* (May 2019), https://www.virtualhospice.ca/en_US/Main+Site+Navigation/Home/Topics/Topics/Final+Days/Children+at+the+Bedside+of+a+Dying+Family+Member+or+Friend.aspx (accessed July 27, 2021).
2. Jessica F. Hinton, "Five Ways to Prepare Young Children to Visit a Loved One Who Is Dying," *Washington Post on Parenting* (July 31, 2018), https://www.washingtonpost.com/news/parenting/wp/2018/07/31/five-ways-to-prepare-young-children-to-visit-a-loved-one-who-is-dying (accessed July 27, 2021).
3. Ira Byock, *The Four Things That Matter Most: A Book about Living*, 10th anniversary edition (New York: Atria Books, 2014).

RECOMMENDED READINGS

III

Unexpected Death and
Associated Concerns

12

⌘

Haunted

Finding Meaning in a Meaningless Death

I listened to the phone message from Joyce, the local nurse. "Hi, Lynne, we had a catastrophe here. A young man, an only child, was killed in a hiking accident. I would like to confer with you, if you can. His mother doesn't want to go to the funeral."

When I returned Joyce's call, she updated me about the mother, Bette: "She has been in bed since she heard the news 24 hours ago. She won't get up, and she won't see anyone."

Three hours later, I entered the yard of the woman's home. Dozens of people were there, friends of Yossi, the deceased. Many were young adults around his age, in their early 20s. Many others were older. People were openly weeping on the road next to the house or speaking in hushed voices; all eyes were red and swollen.

Joyce met me and brought me towards the house. A big man met us on the doorstep: Yossi's father. As we shook hands, he gave me a polite host's smile, clearly happy that I came to see his wife. I didn't feel his grief, only his relief.

I was escorted into a house bursting with people and food. True to our Middle Eastern culture (and many other cultures also), everyone was trying to help "put a bandage on this cancer" with food . . .

I was brought into the hall and stopped. Yossi's girlfriend was ahead of me, the first person Yossi's mother agreed to see. She entered the bedroom. And as I waited in the hall, I began to attract attention. There were many

Clearing the Path. Lynne Dale Halamish and Eric J. Cassell, Oxford University Press. © Lynne Dale Halamish 2022.
DOI: 10.1093/oso/9780197636879.003.0012

people here with whom I had worked before, either as grievers or as professional caregivers. They each greeted me quietly with comments like "It is so good you are here. . . . I wish we didn't need you, but I am so happy to see you here."

I was not comfortable with this recognition, this expectation. I prefer anonymity. I wanted to be quiet and ignored as I prepared myself to enter the room.

Shortly thereafter, the girlfriend left Bette's bedroom, and Joyce went in to tell her that I had come.

The door opened again, and I entered the darkened bedroom. In the half-light I saw a disheveled woman in her early 60s lying in the bed, her arm thrown over her face. The room was small, with no place to sit. I asked and received permission to sit next to her on the bed. She began to cry. I waited silently.

After a few minutes, I asked her what had happened. She looked startled and then began to tell me.

Slowly, with many pauses, I continued to ask quiet, concrete questions. "How did you find out? When? Who told you? What were the words he used? What did you do then?"

"Tell me about Yossi. Who was he? What was he like?" Bette spoke about her son at length, interspersed by crying.

Bette was 42 when Yossi was born—the first successful pregnancy following seven miscarriages. Then at age 6, Yossi almost died from a virulent virus. He was hospitalized for three weeks, teetering on the edge of the chasm, as Bette wailed at the doctors the whole time: "You can't let him die! He's my only child!" And, miraculously, Yossi had lived.

I was astonished. I had worked with numerous families bereaved by this same virus, and I told Bette that I had never heard of a child surviving it. True, many of my clients are bereaved or about to be bereaved; so logically, those who survived would not be seeing me professionally at all. Still, it was amazing that Yossi had survived.

Bette replied that it was because she had refused to let Yossi take antibiotics before the virus; so, when he was ill, the antibiotics were very effective. Medically speaking, viruses are completely unresponsive to antibiotics; but this was her understanding, and I let it pass without challenge.

She then told me that at 18, Yossi went into the army like most Israeli 18-year-olds. But he volunteered for a combat unit, which is unusual for an only child. During his service, he was in both a war and a bad car accident. Again, he escaped death.

Bette said, "The third time is the end."

As we continued speaking, somehow, and I am not sure how, the conversation became focused on how wonderful it was that Bette and her husband had enjoyed Yossi for these 20 years . . . against all those odds. First the late-life conception and normal birth, then the virus at age 6, then the war. I thought to myself, "It is almost as if death has been following this child all his life, and on the fourth attempt, if we count unlikely conception as number one, finally succeeding."

Although musings of this type often seem bizarre, I have learned not to ignore them for two reasons:

1. If I am thinking it, there is at least a chance that the bereaved person may also have entertained the same thought.
2. This specific "bizarre" thought can strangely twist the horror of a situation into a partial victory by providing significance or meaning.

This partial victory does not mean that the grief will disappear, or even be lightened in any way; only that it gives a glimmer of significance. This young man's life was very significant to his mother. His life, in fact, *made* this woman a mother. If all the people milling around outside this room and this house were any indication, Yossi was also significant to others.

The meaning of a given life is very important to most people, including those who weren't close to the deceased. Significance can provide (dare I use the word?) hope here. Perhaps a better way to express it is "an anchor."

For this connection to succeed in bereavement, however, hope must be redefined. "Where there is life, there is hope" is obviously not relevant for the deceased son. But it is relevant perhaps for his mother.

I asked Bette about the funeral, knowing that she had refused to go.

Her response was immediate and as I expected. "I can't go! I *won't* go! Everyone tells me it's important, and that I will regret not going, but I won't regret it."

Every culture has rituals surrounding death. This is because we believe the ritual helps the living in some way. It serves to recognize that a death has occurred, providing a way to be recognized and validated as a mourner, and for the survivors to recognize and adjust to the change in status (from mother to bereaved mother, wife to widow, and so on).

In Bette's culture, the funeral (burial ritual) takes place within 24 to 48 hours—a time too brief to begin to process grief. Processing grief is not the purpose of this ritual; it is rather recognition of the death and the status change of the chief mourners.

Bette's refusal to attend the funeral was a refusal to recognize the death. However, the death has occurred, a reality that separates the living from the deceased. Therefore, its recognition is also necessary: not only that one life has ended, but that other lives are continuing.

"Bette." I waited until her eyes met mine. Then I quietly said, "You need to be there."

"Why? *Why?!* I don't want to!"

"Because no one else can do what you need to do."

"What do I need to do?"

"You need to be his mother there."

"But he's dead!"

"Yes. He is. But you are still his mother. You were his mother from the moment of conception. . . . You must also be his mother at the end. It's abominable that you must bury your child instead of him burying you . . . but no one else can do it."

We sat in silence for a while.

"You have a window of time, Bette. Once he's laid in the ground, that window will close. This can never be redone. This is the only time it can be done."

"I'll go. I'll go!" She said in anger. She threw back her bedcovers and sat up on the bed. "I need water," she murmured as she stood up and went to the door.

Anger, standing, water . . . a much better direction than hiding in bed in a darkened room. Although the path ahead would be riddled with pits and falls, she had begun to walk it.

For the moment, I didn't know if I was being dismissed or if I should follow her. I remained seated. She looked back and waited impatiently.

I stood and accompanied Bette out of the room. We headed for the balcony of her home. We had to walk through the house to get there, passing many of the comforters. They looked at me with admiration, for having "succeeded in getting her out of her room." I avoided eye contact and quickened my pace, uncomfortable with this.

We reached the balcony and found that we were alone there. Bette firmly shut the door behind us.

NOTES TO THE PRACTITIONER

Meaning is very important to most of us—so important that we will create meaning if it is not readily apparent. We may have to look very hard when the circumstances surrounding a death are telling us that the death is meaningless. Unlike a life lost in defending one's country, or while saving others from crime or disaster, the randomness of accidents or other tragedies can seem meaningless. This in turn can appear to rob the life of its significance.

Sometimes finding significance involves assigning meaning, for instance in all of the streets, parks, books, charitable foundations, events, and conferences named "in memory" of deceased persons. Sometimes people join a fight against cancer, against drunk drivers, rescue services, and so on, to be able to assign meaning to a death that seems meaningless.

Generally speaking, when we as counselors hear the background story of a deceased individual, we can often hear meaning that may escape the bereaved storyteller. Often it is only a matter of reflecting this meaning back to the griever, in order for them to see it.

Following trauma, the "noise" inside the traumatized person's head is enormous, with thoughts flying by at breakneck speed. "How could this happen!?" "Is this my fault?" "Why didn't they listen to me?" "What will I do now?" "How can I live with this?" "It's not true!" Losing a loved one feels like a physical beating. Silence, therefore, is an extremely relevant tool here. It provides a supportive presence without additional "static" thrown into the mix.

Throughout this clinical tale, I referred to my feelings of discomfort when approached by others with admiration. When professionals become aware of such an inner response, it should serve as a self-teaching tool: Why did that make me uncomfortable? My answer in this case:

I don't want to be prideful, because it interferes with the work and pushes me towards mistakes. When everyone is lauding you, it is easy to start believing them . . . which hurts your integrity, I think. The discomfort is visceral. It makes me feel like I am wading through mud, and it is hard to maintain clarity. (Personal correspondence with Eric Cassell, January 2018)

CONCLUSIONS

- *Give the stage to the griever. Listen first before offering any opinion; then ask questions that allow the griever to keep the stage.*
- *Allow extended silences, taking into account the deafening internal noise that is present after trauma.*
- *Reinforce the griever's continuing and exclusive role, as mother, husband, son, and so on.*

> • *Search for significance: the importance in attending the funeral, the value of the life that was, and is now no longer, a purpose for the lives that are.*

RECOMMENDED READING

1. Emily Esfahani Smith, "How to Find Meaning in the Face of Death," *The Atlantic: Health* (March 2, 2017), https://www.theatlantic.com/health/archive/2017/03/power-of-meaning/518196/ (accessed July 27, 2021).
2. "Silence in Counselling," *Counselling Tutor*, https://counsellingtutor.com/basic-counselling-skills/silence/ (accessed July 27, 2021).

IV

Funeral-Related Concerns

13

⌒⌒

The Big Event

Children and Family Funerals

"What about the funeral?" Rose asked.

I was on a video call to her hospital room. Her husband, Jacob, sat beside her.

Rose's query surprised me. Usually, it is the healthy spouse who asks about the dying spouse's funeral. However, any question that is raised needs to be addressed.

"Your children should be at the funeral, with someone to accompany each of them individually, in case it's too difficult for Jacob to be with them. Choose someone who is not from the immediate family, but is close to the child and trusted by him or her."

"But," she said quietly, "there's a dilemma."

"What is the dilemma?"

"My family is from a culture where the grieving process often involves screaming, yelling, fainting, and falling on the grave."

"I understand that strong emotional displays can be frightening for children. But it's *their* culture, too. It belongs to them. They simply need to be prepared ahead of time, so that they know what can or will happen. Tell them that it's not dangerous, that it's an expression of feelings, a part of your culture. And seeing that someone will be accompanying each child at the funeral, they will not be dealing with it alone."

I searched the couple's faces to make sure that they were both with me. Then I continued:

Clearing the Path. Lynne Dale Halamish and Eric J. Cassell, Oxford University Press. © Lynne Dale Halamish 2022.
DOI: 10.1093/oso/9780197636879.003.0013

"And Jacob, it's also important for you to tell them, 'There is a strong possibility that I will cry, and that's ok. I will stand up when I need to, and I will cry when I need to.'"

"What if one of the kids says, 'I don't want to go'?" Jacob blurted out.

"First of all, you don't ask them whether or not they want to go. It's a family ceremony. No one has a greater right to be there than Rose's children do. Every culture in the world has some ritual or other surrounding death. We have them because we believe it helps. We want to help your children, don't we?"

I continued: "They will see that many people care about their mother, because there will be many people there. They will see that they are not the only ones who are in pain or miss Rose. They will not feel isolated. They will have a place to mourn instead of being left home, outside of the mourners' circle. Trying to mourn alone can cause great confusion."

I saw Rose silently look into Jacob's face, as his eyes slowly welled up.

I reminded them, "Each of your children will have a trusted adult with them, and they will be given as much information as possible about the funeral ahead of time, including what they are expected to do or how they are expected to act. You can tell them, 'People may cry and scream, and you can also cry or scream if you want to, but you don't have to if you don't want to.'"

"What if the other mourners don't get it?" Rose asked. "What if they say the wrong thing to the kids?"

I smiled and said, "If others know that you consider the children mourners, then they, too, will consider the children mourners, and the children may receive expressions of love and care that they would not have otherwise received. If you do *not* treat the children as mourners, everyone will ignore them, and they will be neglected or marginalized. Children can cope with difficult things if they have enough preparation, if they are told exactly what will happen."

There was a short silence.

"Rose," I said.

"Yes?"

"You really are a hero."

"I hope so." She uttered it quietly.

"Your willingness to look directly at your death, to think about matters of burial, to think about every possible way you can protect your children after you are gone—you are a hero. I hope that when my time comes, I will be a hero like you."

Less than 24 hours after our video call, Jacob called to tell me that Rose had died.

He wanted me to remind him of how to tell the children and what to do at the funeral. We went over all the details.

"So, the funeral is tomorrow?"

"No, it is tonight at 10 pm."

Oh no! If there is one thing that can make a funeral even more difficult and frightening, it's to have it at night! Some religious customs forbid any delay to the burial, so funerals are sometimes scheduled at night out of necessity. But I was dismayed as I remembered the only night funeral I have ever attended.

It was a few years ago. There were spotlights set up at various points in the graveyard. A crowd of people huddled murmuring together, some praying out loud and some speaking softly to each other. As the participants moved towards the open grave, they slowly shuffled into the pools of light and then out again into the night. Because of the spotlights, the shadows of the people were silhouettes on the gravestones as they passed. All were dressed in dark colors. The deceased's body jiggled along on a wheeled stretcher, covered in a black cloth.

After a few seconds, I shook off my memories and reminded myself, "A burial at night is no different from any other burial. And this is also part of their culture."

I reassured Jacob accordingly. "Tell the children that the funeral will be at night," I emphasized. "Tell them there will be spotlights that will create harsh shadows, the way spotlights and flashlights always do. Explain that they are just shadows, and it's okay."

I thought about children's frequent reactions to darkness and moving shadows. What else could help them? Ahh. "Give each of the children a small flashlight of their own to take with them," I suggested.

Still, I felt my heart in my mouth as I uttered this last sentence to him. Despite my conviction that it is important for children to attend family funerals, I felt my own taboo against bringing small children to a night funeral. Sometimes theory and fact are very different. Was my guidance to this family going to prove beneficial or ill-advised?

A few hours after the funeral, I received a message on my phone from Jacob:

"Dear Lynne, the funeral was a good and very significant experience for the children. We will speak later this week. Thank you so much. Jacob."

NOTES TO THE PRACTITIONER

We all prefer the familiar surroundings of our own culture. Our understanding of other cultures is limited, particularly in how they deal with stressful circumstances. Therefore, listening and modifying our own biases is necessary to achieve the optimum outcome for the patient or counselee.

Is there a minimum age that is considered to be proper in dealing with such issues with children? Or does it depend more on the maturity and cognitive ability of the child? A child should be spoken to at the level of their understanding from age 2. But even preverbal children should be included in all family rituals, both joyful and mourning.

It is very important for all immediate family members to attend formal mourning rituals, including children of all ages. If not, they will be sidelined or marginalized, and isolated from the rest of the family during the period when they most need support and inclusion. Their presence at a funeral will also allow them to begin to understand that the death has in fact occurred. These formal mourning rituals exist to assist us, both as adults and as children, to be a part of the communal honoring of the life that has passed.

Knowledge is not necessarily power, but it does tend to serve us well in unknown circumstances. Generally, children have only been exposed to funerals via television or video games, which present a very distorted and sometimes frightening picture. When taking children to a funeral, it is important to clearly describe the most likely scenario that they will be participating in, step by step. This description should include what their role should be. For example: "You will see some people crying. You can cry if you want to, but you don't have to if you don't want to."

CONCLUSIONS

- *All immediate family members, regardless of age, should attend formal mourning rituals.*
- *Children should be prepared ahead of time, both for what will be taking place and how they are expected to act.*
- *Children under 16 should be accompanied by a close friend, who is not an immediate family member, for support.*

RECOMMENDED READING

1. Dougy Center: The National Center for Grieving Children and Families, "Kids and Funerals" (November 2020), https://www.dougy.org/grief-resources/kids-and-funerals/ (accessed July 28, 2021).
2. Mary A. Fristad, Julie Cerel, and Maria Goldman, "The Role of Ritual in Children's Bereavement," *Omega Journal of Death and Dying* 42, no. 4 (2001), https://journ als.sagepub.com/doi/abs/10.2190/MC87-GQMC-VCDV-UL3U (accessed July 28, 2021).

14

⌒∿⌒

It's My Party

Allowing Someone to Speak

Juliet was a theater director. She had a glorious repertoire of plays, concerts, musicals, and holiday shows that she had directed. She was over 80 years old and was suffering from advanced Parkinson's disease.

I was called in by the mental health team in her town. "Juliet is driving everyone crazy!" the caller told me. "You have got to talk to her."

"What is the problem?" I inquired.

"She isn't dying . . . yet. But she *constantly* talks about death. Her husband and kids can't handle it anymore."

Juliet had agreed to talk to me as well. So I made an appointment to see her in her home.

I knocked on her door, "Come in!" she trilled loudly. When I entered, I was greeted by an elderly, overweight woman in a padded recliner with a ventilator attached to her nose. She had a nurse's aide to assist her during the day and was never left alone. Her husband—around the same age, but healthy and younger-looking—had also frequently taken on a care-taking role.

During our one-hour meeting, Juliet dozed off for a minute or two every three to four minutes or so. Strangely, her conscious moments were full of energy between these odd "naps." She explained that this was a result of the medicine she was taking for her disease.

"I understand you asked to see me, Juliet?" I began.

"Yes."

Clearing the Path. Lynne Dale Halamish and Eric J. Cassell, Oxford University Press. © Lynne Dale Halamish 2022.
DOI: 10.1093/oso/9780197636879.003.0014

"How can I help you?"

"Well, I want to direct my funeral, and everyone keeps telling me I'm crazy for wanting to. I can talk to my youngest about it sometimes, but my husband can't stand hearing about it." She paused. "Do *you* think I'm crazy for wanting to plan my own funeral?"

"No, I don't," I replied calmly. "So, Juliet, what do you want at your funeral?"

"Well," she hunkered down in her chair, wiggling her fingers in anticipation. "I would like to speak in the beginning. . . ."

"But you will be dead," I replied, curious about how she would respond to that.

"Yes, of course. I will tape it ahead of time, so everyone can hear me."

"All right, that sounds like a good idea. What next?"

"I want my youngest son to sing a song."

"Is he a good singer?"

"He sings like an angel." She sighed.

"Did you ask him if he would?"

"I did. He said, 'How could I sing right after you die?' "

"And . . .?"

"Well, I told him we would tape that part, too." I looked at her as she gathered her thoughts and continued: "Then, I want my daughter-in-law to read all the things I have done, my personal history, to the mourners at the cemetery."

"Do you want to hear what she will say ahead of time?" I asked.

"Absolutely!"

"Does she agree?"

"She will," she replied confidently.

"Okay, then what?"

"Then everyone goes home."

"So, where would you like to be buried? Do you want to be dressed in specific clothing or a shroud?"

"It will be in the town cemetery. A shroud will be fine."

"Do you want to be an organ donor?"

"No."

"When would you like to die?"

"After this is all taken care of."

"So, are you thinking of committing suicide?"

"Oh, no!" She looked shocked at the question. "Of course not!"

"Okay. Good." I had to make sure. "So, *how* would you like to die?"

"Painlessly." She had obviously thought that part through already.

"Are you in pain right now?"

"No, the drugs prescribed to me are taking care of the pain."

"So, you trust the doctors to manage your pain?"

"Yes. I also trust the nurses."

"Good." I paused for a minute.

"So, Juliet, I suggest that you write down your plan, record your speech, ask your son to record the song. Ask your daughter-in-law to write the history. Clearly label everything and their order in the funeral. Put it all in a drawer and let your husband know where it is. Then you can stop talking about it, because it will all be settled."

Juliet responded with a roar of laughter. "Very good!"

Then, she asked me in a more serious tone, "Why do you think it's so important to me to have this all planned out?"

"Because you're a control freak," I answered candidly, with a smile. "But that's fine."

"That's right, I am! Always have been." She was smiling again, and she looked like a weight had been lifted off her shoulders. She was even breathing more deeply.

"Is there anything else I can do for you?" I asked.

"No, I just needed your authorization that I'm not crazy. And that I can do this."

"You've got it," I replied.

As I left Juliet's home, I met with the mental health director and explained that Juliet's talk of her not-quite-so-imminent death was not problematic; she simply had an unusual hands-on approach to the event. And to remove any doubt, I added that I had helped her map out her plan.

NOTES TO THE PRACTITIONER

Dreams, desires, fears, and anxieties can rob us of our sleep and peace of mind. Verbalizing these things is known as the "talking cure"; it is the basis of counseling. Writing these troubling thoughts down, even (and often primarily) those things that we are afraid to say aloud, can give us some breathing space from their intrusive pressure. For example, consider a parent feeling tremendous guilt for having anticipatory thoughts about their sick child's funeral. They may feel that such thoughts are traitorous, perhaps even that they could compromise the child's chances of healing. However, these thoughts are in fact very prevalent among parents of seriously ill children.

The remedy is quite simple. When someone is suffering from intrusive or unwanted thoughts or worries, advise them to write down what they want or fear, put the page in a safe place, and then they can stop thinking about it constantly and go on with their lives. Make sure, however, that their thoughts are not putting themselves or anyone else at risk of harm.

The case described here was quite clear. It is not "crazy" that an 80-year-old woman with a proactive personality would want to plan her own funeral. The most reasonable response is to listen and help her to plan it as much as possible. As long as she is not suicidal, there is no problem with her planning her "final performance."

CONCLUSIONS

- *Despite the reality that nothing in life is more certain than dying, the taboo against talking about it will frequently cause caretakers to be alarmed if patients wish to discuss their own funeral arrangements.*
- *Generally, persistent talk about the end of one's own life signifies a need for someone to listen and discuss these issues.*
- *The practitioner or counselor can give a sense of control to someone feeling anxiety about this event, by helping the person to identify and record his or her preferences about the circumstances.*

RECOMMENDED READING

1. Mariana Plata, "How to Listen to Someone Without Judgment," *Psychology Today* online (July 7, 2020), https://www.psychologytoday.com/intl/blog/the-gen-y-psy/202007/how-listen-someone-without-judgment (accessed July 28, 2021).
2. Marie Curie, "Care and Support Through Terminal Illness" (February 5, 2021), https://www.mariecurie.org.uk/professionals/palliative-care-knowledge-zone/individual-needs/talking-approaching-end-life (accessed July 28, 2021).

V

After Death

Bereavement-Related Concerns

15

✦

Clearing the Path

Holding on by Letting Go

Naphtali, an active soldier in his early 20s, came to see me. It had been two years since the death of his mother.

"I barely spent any time with her during her illness, before she passed. I was in the middle of training for a special elite unit, and I didn't get much time off. I don't think I was paying attention. . . . I was able to visit her right before she passed, to say goodbye, but that was all. At the time I was still in training, so I didn't see my family much, or help them either. Only now, two years later, I started thinking that there might be something wrong with me, because I was so detached from it all. Can you help me, or is it too late? Have I damaged myself permanently by not coming sooner?"

"Not at all," I said. "This is not an emergency. Saying goodbye to your mother was time-sensitive, and you were able to accomplish that. This is not time-sensitive."

I continued: "This is actually the dilemma that combat soldiers face. It's like being in the foxhole on the front line of a battle. When a fellow soldier is suddenly killed, you cannot stop and mourn him, or you, too, might be killed. You must wait to grieve until you're in a safe place again. In your case, you were stationed on two demanding fronts simultaneously, both before and after your mother passed: your intensive military training and your family's trauma. You needed to wait for a safe space to deal with her death personally."

Clearing the Path. Lynne Dale Halamish and Eric J. Cassell, Oxford University Press. © Lynne Dale Halamish 2022.
DOI: 10.1093/oso/9780197636879.003.0015

"No additional damage is caused by waiting to grieve. Some people come to me decades after losing someone to deal with their grief. Suspended grief behaves a lot like fresh bread stored in the freezer. No matter when it's defrosted, it's still fresh. The only problem is your environment. You won't receive the support mourners usually get from those around them, because of all the time gone by since your mother's death. The people around you will not attribute your feelings to grief—they'll assume you're already past that."

I paused to let him respond. His thinking had meanwhile taken a different direction.

"I am holding onto her . . . my mom . . . as tightly as I can." He said this with determination, his eyes fixed on his boots.

"What do you mean?" I inquired.

"Any object I have of hers, any sadness I feel, I really hold onto it."

"Okay. I want to explain something about grief," I said. "You don't need to hold onto it. I understand that it feels like you're holding onto your mother. But, Naphtali, the grief you feel is *not her*."

"What do you mean?" He sounded perplexed.

"When did the grief come for the first time, before you froze it?" I asked.

"When she died."

"Not *when* she died. *After* she died."

"What?" Naphtali looked even more confused than before.

"That's what shows that the grief is 100% *not* your mother. It only came after she died. You won't win back any piece of your mother by holding onto grief."

I waited a moment until he had thought this through and returned his eyes to me. "It's actually the opposite. The more you let go of the grief, the more of your mother you will get back again."

"But . . . I thought my sadness keeps her close."

I was firm as I continued, "No. Your sadness, your grief for your mother is like a wall between you and her. You can't see her or feel her when it's strong, only when it begins to fall away. I know this is not what logic might tell you, but it's very true. Ending the grief process does not mean erasing your mother. It does not mean forgetting her. It does not mean never missing her again."

Now he was curious. "So, what *does* it mean?"

"Ending the grief means choosing to take down the wall. You come to accept your new relationship with her. In time, it means wanting to smile when her memory comes to mind, instead of weeping or feeling miserable."

"Most people are not aware of this," I continued, "but in my experience, releasing the grief makes it possible to heal the wound made by the separation. The grief process also has a purpose and needs to happen. It can't be done quickly, but don't hold onto it any longer than you have to."

In our final meeting, Naphtali mentioned that the most helpful pieces of information were two of the subjects we had discussed: finding out that he was not damaged by delaying grief, and learning that he didn't have an obligation to hold onto grief indefinitely.

NOTES TO THE PRACTITIONER

In his iconic work, *A Grief Observed*, C. S. Lewis wrote about his surprise in discovering life after bereavement:

"Something quite unexpected has happened. It came this morning early. For various reasons, not in themselves at all mysterious, my heart was lighter than it had been for many weeks. . . . The sun was shining and there was a light breeze. And suddenly at the very moment when, so far, I mourned [my wife] least, I remembered her best. Indeed, it was something (almost) better than memory; an instantaneous, unanswerable impression. To say it was like a meeting would be going too far. Yet there was that in it which tempts one to use those words. It was as if the lifting of the sorrow removed a barrier. Why has no one ever told me these things?"

One of the valuable tools available to assist those in treatment is normalization. When patients come to you, fearful that they have contracted a disease, and it turns out they haven't, you reassure them to relieve them of the anxiety associated with the disease. The same is true following trauma, bad news, or death in a family.

Since speaking about death is generally taboo in Western society, most people in that culture are not aware of what normal grief looks like. Therefore, normalization is a big part of grief counseling, medicine, and psychology.

People who have been living in the shadow of serious illness are in a perpetual state of tension, ready to jump into action in case a medical crisis arises. That tension is no longer needed after the death of the ill loved one, and the grievers need reassurance that they can relax as they grieve. "There is no emergency now. Breathe when you can. Take your time."

They also need to know that grief can be a long process. Grief doesn't get resolved in days, or even weeks, as is the general expectation; we usually speak in terms of years (1–5 years, depending on the relationship and other factors). But it can be *finite*.

Thus, the goal of grief counseling is threefold:
1. Normalization
2. Reassurance
3. Helping the mourner avoid pathology, including chronic grief

CONCLUSIONS

- *A big part of grief counseling is normalization. Therefore, it is important for health and mental health practitioners to be aware of normal and abnormal paths of grief.*
- *Many people confuse holding onto grief with holding onto the deceased loved one. It is important to let them know that releasing the grief will give them a closer connection to their loved one than holding onto the grief.*
- *Grieving is not an emergency. It is an open-ended process.*

RECOMMENDED READING

1. Sally A. Dominick, A. Blair Irvine, Natasha Beauchamp, John Steeley, et al., "An Internet Tool to Normalize Grief," *Omega (Westport)* 60, no. 1 (2009): 71–87, https://www.ncbi.nlm.nih.gov/pmc/articles/PMC2802222/ (accessed July 28, 2021).
2. Carol DerSarkissian, "What Is Normal Grieving, and What Are the Stages of Grief?," *Web MD* (November 9, 2020), https://www.webmd.com/balance/normal-grieving-and-stages-of-grief (accessed July 28, 2021).

16

⚜

Refresh

Neutralizing Destructive Memorials

Martha brought her 22-year-old son, Ben, to see me. After a short discussion, it became clear that due to posttraumatic stress (either caused or aggravated by his army service), he was dangerously suicidal. I looked at them both and addressed Ben directly: "You are sick, and you need something I cannot provide. Please go and meet with a psychiatrist for help."

This was my only meeting with Ben.

Several years later, I received a call from Martha asking to meet with me. She reminded me that we had met with her son several years previously, and that I had referred them to a psychiatrist. She also informed me that eventually he did commit suicide.

We set up an appointment, but I was a bit bewildered by her desire to meet me again. Perhaps she wanted to talk about that one meeting that we had so long ago. Perhaps she was coming to blame me for Ben's death.

When she came to the clinic, I asked her why she wanted to meet. She started her answer by relating what had happened since our first meeting.

"During the course of Ben's illness, I left no stone unturned, traditional or alternative. I went everywhere and tried everything to save him. After his death, I continued to try everything to deal with his death. But nothing has worked. I haven't had a good night's sleep for years."

She looked down at her hands in her lap. "So, I decided to come to you."

Clearing the Path. Lynne Dale Halamish and Eric J. Cassell, Oxford University Press. © Lynne Dale Halamish 2022.
DOI: 10.1093/oso/9780197636879.003.0016

I asked her to tell me about Ben, who he was. I heard the story of his illness, which had gone on for a long while. I listened to the details of his eating disorder and her attempts to save him. She described a loving, sweet son, "taken over by a monster"—her words for his crippling psychological problem.

In subsequent meetings, we began the grueling work of saying goodbye to Ben. I guided her to write letters to him. One letter was her homework for every session: "Forgive me," "I forgive you," "I love you," "Thank you," and finally, "Goodbye."

After reading me the third letter, she told me about another side effect of Ben's disease: horrible communication. The loving son had sent hundreds of hate-filled, accusatory text messages and letters to his mother throughout the years of his illness.

I asked her what had become of those. She told me that they were still on her phone. She read a few of them aloud to me: "You are a horrible mother. I hate you!"; "I had always been ashamed of you"; "I wish you were dead!"

"Why do you keep them?" I asked her.

Martha's sad but resolute answer: "They are all I have left of him."

I then told her a story. It was about a 5-year-old boy whose father had died from a painful illness. During the formal mourning period, he came to his mother who sat in a corner weeping, took one of her hands in both of his small hands, and said, "Mom, I know it's sad that Dad has died, but think of the good side." His mother asked, bewildered, "What is the good side?" And her son said, "When he died, the terrible disease that he had died, too."

Martha sat in wonder. "What a lovely story," she said.

"Yes, Martha, it is," I agreed. "You, on the other hand, have kept your son's disease alive, long after it took him away from you—and ruined your own life for years. Those messages are the psychological disorders talking. That's not your son talking. The text messages you read to me don't sound *anything* like who you said your son really was."

She looked startled; the distinction was clearly a new idea to her.

I continued, "You need to erase those text messages, get rid of those letters, and bury the illness that buried your son."

Martha thought for a moment. "Okay . . . I think I can do that."

"Good. Take out your cell phone."

She looked like a deer caught in headlights for a few seconds. Then slowly, reluctantly, she cooperated.

"Open the last message that you read to me. The one Ben wrote the day he died."

She did.

"Erase it."

"I'll erase it later."

This is why she came to me, I thought to myself. "You need support when you do it. Erase it now."

Her finger trembled as it reached out and tapped the "Delete" button.

I asked her, "How many of these messages do you have?"

"Maybe a hundred . . . maybe more."

"Then this was only the first. Erase the others at home."

We concluded the meeting and scheduled another for two weeks later.

As she walked in for our next meeting, I immediately noticed that she was standing straight for the first time since I met her. She looked me in the eyes rather than staring at her feet. She gave me a shy smile.

"How are you, Martha?"

"Better . . . now."

"Talk to me."

"When I left you last time, I went to my car and felt sick because I had erased Ben's message. I cried. I started to drive home. But then I stopped by the side of the road, and I began erasing message after message. When I got home, I had a fever and I started vomiting. I went to bed and slept for six hours straight, till my husband woke me up because he was worried. We had dinner together and then we both went to sleep. I slept deeply through the entire night—and when I woke up, I was better. I feel now like there's some hope. A way out."

I explained to her about the influence the soul can have on the body. "Martha, you were sick because you became addicted to the illness, the guilt, and the pain. What you experienced after erasing those messages was withdrawal."

She thought for a moment and then she replied, "Somehow I knew I would get sick if I came to you, but I thought you might help."

We sat silently for a while. I then added a thought:

"You know, in the Middle Ages, one of the punishments for murder was to chain the body of the victim to his murderer's back, until the corpse would rot and infect the murderer with some disease that eventually killed him. It's as though you chained your son's killer to your back, and you were carrying it around for a long time while it was killing you. Erasing those messages was unlocking those chains."

She looked at me in surprise. "Yes. That is exactly how I feel. I could never have said it myself, but that is exactly what happened."

After a moment, I made another suggestion. "I believe it would be a good idea to walk around your home and yard, look at each thing in it and decide if they are 'clean' or part of Ben's sickness. Get rid of the sickness trash.

Gather it into garbage bags and take it out of your house. Reclaim your living space with your footsteps."

She left me gratefully, even euphoric, and determined to apply this idea.

Two months later, Martha gave me a final update. "Once the prison door had opened," she said, "and the chains fell off my wrists and ankles, I just stood there . . . free, but with no idea which direction to go. I decided to go back to school, and start over in a new direction, a new life. I'm fed up with just existing—I choose to live."

NOTES TO THE PRACTITIONER

Following the death of a loved one, our tendency is to try to hold onto that person. This attempt frequently drives us to cherish objects that were theirs: photographs, letters, clothing, songs, artwork, or other things they created. They may also include favorite places, foods, and friends of theirs that we couldn't tolerate while the loved one was alive . . . anything that will let us think we are keeping a part of the departed life.

Sometimes these serve as "transitional objects" to help us through the grief. Other times, as seen in the story here, they are destructive and prevent us from returning to healthy life. This subject is discussed in more depth in Chapter 19, "Renovation."

In the throes of immediate grief, we may also see a tendency to display large photographs of the deceased; these are very easy to hang up but extremely difficult to remove.

CONCLUSIONS

- *Mourners can become confused between healthy and unhealthy memorabilia.*
- *On the one hand, it is good to cherish reminders of the best things about the deceased person.*
- *On the other hand, it is dangerous to glorify or build up the deceased person in our minds, because everyone else comes out poorly by comparison.*
- *In many families, as in Martha's, but not specifically referred to in this story, there are other children in the family. An obsession with the deceased child can destroy relationships with the live children.*

RECOMMENDED READING

1. Richard D. Goldstein, Carter R. Petty, Sue E. Morris, Melanie Human, Hein Odendaal, et al., "Transitional Objects of Grief," *Comprehensive Psychiatry* 98 (April 2020), https://www.sciencedirect.com/science/article/pii/S0010440X2 0300031 (accessed July 29, 2021).
2. Nadia Khan, "What Is Repetitive Compulsion and How to Overcome It," February 15, 2021, https://www.betterhelp.com/advice/personality-disorders/ what-is-repetitive-compulsion-how-to-overcome-it/ (accessed July 29, 2021).

17

⌇

Hand-Me-Down Death

Blessing and Cursing

L eah, a 45-year-old woman who had been bereaved of her mother 4 years ago, came into my clinic accompanied by her husband, Robert.

She was dressed in a sweatsuit and wore no make-up. Her hair was pulled into a rough ponytail, and her undyed hair roots were showing. Robert began narrating their story, without any response or participation from Leah. The whole time her husband was talking, she herself seemed absent.

The couple admitted that she was only coming to me at Robert's urging. For the past 4 years, he had been taking her to many different types of therapists and counselors—both conventional and nonconventional—but Leah could not find relief from her grief.

When Robert paused in his narrative, I turned to Leah and quietly asked about her mother. She responded slowly, like a rusty gate, as if her voice was scratchy from disuse. Her recital became gradually smoother, and she began to make eye contact.

"My mother was slowly dying for about 12 years. During that time, she told me, and . . ." She paused and met my eyes for the first time. "Throughout my life, she used to tell me that she can't die; because if she dies, I die."

She looked down at her hands. "We were so close; I loved her very much."

"What does it mean, 'if she dies, you will die'?"

Robert sat up and opened his mouth to explain. I lifted my hand to stop him, never taking my eyes off of Leah.

"Since she has died, I feel like my life is over."

Clearing the Path. Lynne Dale Halamish and Eric J. Cassell, Oxford University Press. © Lynne Dale Halamish 2022.
DOI: 10.1093/oso/9780197636879.003.0017

"Because . . .?"

"I never dress up, wear make-up, or go out for fun anymore. I feel like I have died. But I have to keep on; because if I die, my children will die."

"Your children will die . . ." As I echoed her words, my mind was racing. An intergenerational curse? Is there such a thing? How did that play out in the family relationships?

"Yes."

"Have you ever said that to your children?"

"Oh yes, I say it all the time."

Her husband chimed in: "Leah used to be so fun and happy, and she has completely changed since her mother died."

A witness. This significant change was not her imagination.

"Not only that," Robert continued, "but her mother's mother, Leah's grandmother, always said to her own daughter: 'If I die, you will die.' In fact, in the old country, when Leah's mother was only 5 years old, she saw her mother fall through the ice of a frozen pond, and she—at age 5!—jumped right in after her. Not to save her, but to die with her. They were both rescued by a farmer who happened to pass by."

I turned to Leah for confirmation. She nodded, and I summed up what I had just heard.

"Over the past 15 minutes, you have repeatedly stated that your mother was afraid to die because she claimed that you would die with her if she did. You also said that you need to keep living because *your* children would die with *you*. Robert, your husband, has said that your grandmother told your mother repeatedly that *she* would die if your *grandmother* died."

I waited for her confirmation as she nodded and went on to summarize her nonverbal signals. "You say all of these things, confirm all this with a sense of pride and some resignation, as if it were a sign of something essential and positive."

Leah had no problem agreeing with that. "Yes, it is. It shows how much we loved each other," she said, with a bit more enthusiasm than she had shown up to this point.

"Leah, this is not the positive thing you think it is. It's not a blessing; it is, in fact, a curse. It's just like the ancient biblical curses that got passed down through generations."

Now she *did* have a problem. She looked bewildered.

"Can you use words like 'curse' in therapy?"

I explained. "I am telling you what I see. This isn't about spells, or bad-luck signs. We as human beings influence others with our words, our evaluations of their worth, and our predictions for their future.

"What are the fundamental identifying characteristics of blessing and cursing? When we 'predict' life, abundance, meaning and longevity, we are blessing. When we forecast death, emptiness, and meaninglessness, we are cursing." *

"Whether we realize it or not, our declaration of a blessing or a curse on someone has the power to promote life or death."

"In your family, a death curse on a child with the mother's death has gone through three generations. Your grandmother, probably unintentionally, cursed your mother. Your mother, perhaps innocently, passed this on and cursed you. And you. . . . You have already cursed your own children."

Leah's shock showed on her face, and she started to protest. "But I *love* my children!"

I continued, "I'm sure you do. This curse has nothing to do with lack of love. It's possible that your mother loved you very much. She may have shown it in many different ways. This prediction was just not one of them. Do not confuse a curse with a blessing, just because it came from a loved one."

How *do* we differentiate between declarations that curse and those that bless? It's not as straightforward as it seems.

What did I observe in Leah's case? Her mother's declaration gave her no choice at all; only a sense of inevitability as her mother's death approached. And when that death occurred, the curse began to "come true." I saw a formerly vital woman disappearing. I saw someone who felt that she no longer had the right to live. I saw a mother who believed that her own death would likewise end the lives of her children.

I spoke to Leah briefly about the cost of this curse in her life, her children's lives, and potential future generations.

She understood.

We sat in silence. I waited for Leah to meet my eyes with hers before I continued.

"You need to break this curse. For your children. For yourself."

Again, I waited for her to collect herself. She finally took a deep breath and looked up from her hands. So I went on.

"I would like to suggest some practical steps that you can take to break the hold these statements have on you. Would that be acceptable to you?"

---

* This concept is embedded in ancient wisdom, such as Deuteronomy 30:19: "I call heaven and earth as witnesses to you today, that I have set before you life and death, blessing and cursing; therefore, choose life, that both you and your descendants may live."

הללקהו הכרבה ךינפל יתתנ תומהו םייחה הארק ךתא םויה ץרַאה תאו םימשה תא ךב יתדיעה
:ךיערזו התא היחת ןעמל םייחב תרחבו

She said she would be willing to listen.

"First of all, write a letter to your deceased mother. In this letter, you can list any or all of the things you have been thinking about for the past 4 years, since her death. It's also important to write that you forgive her for cursing you by passing this statement on to you, and teaching you to pass it on to your children.

"You can write something like this: 'I know you received this curse from your mother and passed it on to me. It has cost me 4 years of my life so far, but I am not willing to keep paying for this family curse. I am not willing to pass it on to my children and grandchildren. I am choosing to forgive you for this curse. I know you mistakenly took it for a blessing, and I forgive you.'"

I intentionally spoke slowly and clearly, avoiding unnecessary words or any additional material that would clutter the message. I waited for the ideas to settle, and for her confirmation that she had heard and was considering this.

"This next point is essential. That curse has become an automatic thought. Every time you repeated it, you validated it. The curse has become part of your mental repertoire. In order to break this cycle, it is vital that you *stop* repeating it. It will keep ringing in your head for a long time, and after that it will come less often, but as an intrusive thought. Whenever you hear this thought, you need to reject it out loud."

In the same way that she had confirmed the curse, she would need to counter it: verbally. Out of her mouth and in through both her ears.

"For example, your response can be: 'What? That's ridiculous. Children don't die because their parents have died. It is the natural way of life for parents to die *before* their adult children do.' You don't have to believe it in order to say it. Just as the curse was repeated to you until you believed it, its opposite must be repeated until you break free from its power. This is something you need to repeat like clockwork, every time the thought comes."

"Next—put on some make-up and a nice dress, and go out with your husband, at least once a week."

She looked at me, startled, and said, "I can't get dressed up and go out. I can't enjoy myself."

"Don't tell me you can't. You can, Leah. If you *won't*, then that's another story. You don't have to enjoy yourself, at least not at first. Just do it."

She glanced over at Robert, then back at me, and nodded slightly.

"And finally, meet with your children and tell them that what you have been repeating is not true. Of course they won't die if you die first."

A week later, Leah came back to my clinic. I barely recognized her.

She was sporting a stylish new haircut with some colorful highlights. She wore a sharp outfit and make-up. But the most arresting aspects of her change were her posture and her smile.

She told me that she had written the letter and had started fighting the intrusive thoughts. She read the letter to me, and then looked up and smiled. She could tell—as I also could—that she had turned a corner.

However, she couldn't yet bring herself to speak with her children about the destructive statements that had passed from one generation to another, to finally land on them.

As a solution, she asked if she could bring the children in for a meeting with me. I agreed, on the condition that Leah and her husband would be present. Their presence is imperative in a session of this type. It will confirm their agreement with what is being said, and it will eliminate any possibility of "secrets" surrounding the subject.

A week later, I met with the whole family. The children didn't know why they were there. I explained that we wanted to set a few things straight. I then asked if there were any kids in their school whose parents had died.

Michelle, a 13-year-old, volunteered that there was a girl in her class, Yael, whose mom had died 2 months earlier. I asked her how the girl was doing.

She said, "Well, she's kind of sad . . . but sometimes she's just like the rest of us."

I asked, "Will Yael die because her mom died?"

Michelle promptly answered, "Of course not."

I asked her why not, and she replied that kids don't die because their parents die. I told her that this is absolutely correct, and that she is a bright child.

Her brother James, aged 8 and in the third grade, said with surprise: "They don't?"

Everyone in the room looked at him, a bit startled.

"Of course not," Michelle and I both replied in unison and laughed. Leah and I exchanged meaningful looks over the heads of the family.

Michelle turned to her brother and explained: "Kids are *supposed to* live longer than their parents."

NOTES TO THE PRACTITIONER

Today, even the words *blessing* and *curse* evoke images from antiquated cultures. Western societies regard them as either metaphorical expressions or superstition. However, words do have impact, depending on who is saying them to whom, and from what age or in what situation they are uttered.

As we see in this narrative, some blessings or curses can have a very powerful and even a life-altering effect on someone who is vulnerable to them. Besides parents, any health professional who is functioning as an authority figure, such as a physician, nurse, officer, or psychologist, needs to be aware of the possible impact of the spoken or written word on the hearer. We *can* bless them, just as we would certainly like to be blessed by those around us.

During the meetings I spent with the couple in this narrative, one of the tasks I assigned them was to dress up and go out. Directions that work towards reconnecting with life following a loss of life are significant. The goal is not enjoyment, although that can be a byproduct. The goal is reentering the stream of life.

CONCLUSIONS

- *Listening carefully is vital to discovering misconceptions.*
- *Misconceptions or statements carried from our childhood can become ingrained thoughts.*
- *One way to discourage or deflate these thoughts is by repeatedly challenging them out loud.*

RECOMMENDED READING

1. John Preston, "Destructive Thinking: Can You Stop the Cycle?," January 11, 2012, https://athealth.com/topics/destructive-thinking-can-you-stop-the-cycle/ (accessed July 29, 2021).
2. Rebecca Joy Stanborough, "How to Change Negative Thinking with Cognitive Restructuring," February 4, 2020, https://www.healthline.com/health/cognitive-restructuring (accessed July 29, 2021).

18

❧

The Taj Mahal

Choosing to Leave Your Ghosts Behind

Bob had lost his wife to COVID-19. It was quite sudden. She woke up one morning with what seemed like a bad case of the flu. Two days later, she was dead . . . leaving him to raise two small girls on his own.

We met for about 6 months. Bob spoke about their house and children as if they were hers, never "ours" or "mine." It was disturbing—almost as if *he* had died and *she* had survived.

In widowhood situations, the survivor can often make the home theirs by changing the interior, either partially or significantly. When the house remains exactly the same, filled with reminders of the deceased, it is very challenging to move on. As long as everything was hers and nothing was his, he would not be able to turn away from death towards life.

"Move to a new house," I advised.

"I can't, I can't leave her house," Bob pleaded. "I can't leave *her*."

"You didn't leave her. *She* left *you*."

"She didn't choose to." Bob sighed deeply as his eyes glazed over.

"No," I agreed. "But she *did* leave you. And your girls."

I waited for his response. He bowed his head and looked at his hands.

"Bob," I asked, "where do you see yourself 10 years from now?"

"What? I can't see myself at all without her."

"But, Bob, you already *are* without her." I paused and then went on. "Ten years down the road, do you want to be alone?"

Clearing the Path. Lynne Dale Halamish and Eric J. Cassell, Oxford University Press. © Lynne Dale Halamish 2022.
DOI: 10.1093/oso/9780197636879.003.0018

Bob lifted his eyes towards the ceiling with a small sniffle. It may have been the first time since his wife's passing that he thought of himself as "alone."

"No," he finally replied. "But it's too soon. It's only been 6 months."

"I'm not asking you about today. I'm asking you about a choice."

This is a deliberate challenge that is often effective. It involves shifting the survivor's focus away from death and helping them choose life. It is a process that begins with the head (making a choice) and ends with the feet (taking affirmative action). Grief is a forked road. The griever may stand still at the junction for a long time, but you can help them start to slowly turn towards life, one step at a time.

"What choice are you talking about?" Bob looked at me.

"The choice to live. Being alone can become a habit, and over time that can become hard to break. Right now, you only need to make a choice. For *your*-self. For *your* girls."

Three months later (now 9 months after his wife's death), Bob came back to meet me again.

"So, have you spent time with anyone?" I inquired. "Seen anyone that you could be interested in?"

"No. It feels like a betrayal. She is my wife."

"She *was* your wife, Bob. Your marriage was an agreement to be partners until death parts you. Death has parted you."

"I've tried going on a few dates, but I can't bring another woman into her house."

I leaned forward, towards him, and looked earnestly into his eyes: "Move."

"I can't sell this house. The house is hers."

"You need to move, in order to live. Your children deserve at least one living parent. You have turned their home into a memorial."

He suddenly seemed excited. "Yes! Like the pyramids. Like the Taj Mahal." Bob smiled enthusiastically. "All symbols of a great, undying love!"

"Indeed," I replied, "and all of them are graves. None of them are places of life. Beauty and love on the outside—death and bare bones on the inside. No one can live in a graveyard, or should have to. Not you, and not your children."

A heavy silence fell on the small room.

"You know what?" I added, a few moments later. "Don't sell the house. Rent it out, and rent another place for you and the children to live in."

"I can't let anyone else live here. It's *her* house."

I thought for a moment. "Can you afford to rent a place for yourself and the children, and leave your house empty?"

He mulled it over for a while, and then said, "I could do it for a few months."

"Do it," I said, "and see how it feels. While you're there, try to pay attention. Watch your children. Observe their behavior, as well as your own. Is it better or worse? Easier or harder? Is it difficult to breathe, or does the air have more oxygen?"

They rented an apartment in the same neighborhood, so that the girls wouldn't have to change schools.

When we spoke again, a couple months later, Bob reported that he felt lighter . . . but also somewhat guilt-ridden. The children, however, definitely seemed livelier. They didn't talk about their old house. They didn't ask to go back, not even to visit.

After a while, Bob met a friend. The friendship budded into a relationship. She moved into the rented home with Bob and his girls.

After 3 more months, he started renting out "her" house.

And 6 months after that, Bob and his new partner bought a new house together. A short time later, they added a baby boy of their own to the family.

Bob finally sold the old house.

One step at a time, he had chosen life, for himself and for his children.

NOTES TO THE PRACTITIONER

Only three types of death change the mourner's status in a way that makes it more challenging to reach the end of the mourning period:

1. Losing an only child, which can strip the parent of their mother/father status.
2. Losing both parents, turning the child into an orphan.
3. Losing a spouse, making the griever a widow/er.

As the story demonstrates, someone who was part of a couple—a team—and now is not can feel lost. If most of their friends are also couples, the widow/er becomes a third wheel in social situations. If the couple was mostly together without others in their life, the widow/er will have to fill the void. This need to find new friends comes just at the most vulnerable point in their life, when they don't have the strength to find them.

Another overwhelming change is household management. The couple probably divided the household tasks between them, as many couples do. The survivor may not be familiar with either the scope or the type of functions their departed spouse used to fill, until they are confronted by tasks going undone. Their income may be reduced, they might be unable to sleep alone, and many other new issues may come to the forefront. If there are young children in the family, suddenly the new widow/er will have to make all the decisions concerning them without the former partner. They will experience all the resulting pains and joys as a single parent.

Finally, there are the inner challenges. Widowhood forces the left-behind spouse to redefine themselves: Who are they as a single person? How much of their behavior was modified by being part of a couple? Which habits are their own, and which would they rather not keep?

If the home is filled with reminders of the dead, it can often become a place where life cannot continue. The house becomes a memorial to the past, "haunted" by the objects that belonged to the deceased. It can become uncomfortable for other people to visit, further isolating the bereaved.

The earlier the griever decides to go on living, the better. This can happen within the first few hours, days, or weeks. If it doesn't, the decision to live can still be made afterward, but it will involve breaking the newly acquired habit of living with a "ghost" rather than connecting with other living people. It is better, albeit harder, to choose life at the time of death, or as close as possible to that time.

Choosing to live does not necessarily involve a task, only a conscious decision. Deciding to live doesn't depend on feelings. The decision is not betrayal or abandonment of the departed loved one, although many may feel guilty about it. It is often effective to point out that the survivor is not leaving the deceased behind; the deceased spouse is the one who effectively left the relationship, regardless of whether or not they chose to leave.

CONCLUSIONS

- *Widowhood involves redefining oneself, which is often a labor-intensive process.*
- *The decision to live following the death of a loved one is necessary to reconnect with life.*
- *Sometimes, such a decision involves reclaiming territory for the living, or moving to a new location to escape the "tomb."*

RECOMMENDED READING

1. "Making an active decision to live after horrible trauma is often the first step to recovery, even while the aftershocks of the trauma are still fresh. If we wait too long to make this decision, our 'nondecision' can solidify and become difficult to identify and break out of." From L. Halamish and D. Hermoni, "Deciding to Live," in *The Weeping Willow: Encounters with Grief* (New York: Oxford University Press, 2007), 60–61.
2. Richard Ballo, "Seven Ways to Come Back to Life After Suffering the Death of a Loved One" [blog], https://richardballo.com/seven-ways-to-come-back-to-life-after-suffering-the-death-of-a-loved-one/ (accessed August 4, 2021).

19

Renovation

Reframing the Narrative

Rachel was a 51-year-old widow. She had been married to her husband Leonard for 6 years, when he killed himself. This was 12 years before our meeting.

I asked her to tell me her story.

"It was his second marriage, my first. I adored him. He was an artist, a gifted photographer, a pure soul, a wonderful and amazing man. He loved his art, and I loved him. He never worked for a living. I supported us. But . . .

"I received no remuneration for it in care, tenderness, or thanks. I was barren and wanted children so badly. He had three children from his first wife, so he wouldn't allow me to get fertility treatments. He was an outstanding photographer. He made a twice-life-sized painting of his pregnant first wife and hung it up in our home."

Despite the difficult situation Rachel was describing, during our meeting she never ceased her worshipful attitude towards Leonard, or her conviction that she was the fortunate one to have had him as a spouse. It even appeared as if she was grateful for the large photograph of his first wife hanging in their home.

"Twelve years ago, he killed himself by jumping off the top of a tall building. He left no note. Leonard's family, with whom I had so far had a decent relationship, blamed me for his suicide and ended all contact with me. Even for his annual memorial . . . I am not invited and unwanted. It was easy for them to dismiss me. He had always been verbally harsh with

Clearing the Path. Lynne Dale Halamish and Eric J. Cassell, Oxford University Press. © Lynne Dale Halamish 2022.
DOI: 10.1093/oso/9780197636879.003.0019

me, regardless of the presence of others. But I was lucky to have him as a husband."

When speaking of the treatment she received at the hands of Leonard's relatives, her tone and manner were pained and she teared up. I remained silent for the moment.

Rachel was 32 when she married Leonard. Until 6 months before the wedding, she had thought that she would never marry, and she was desperate to have a family. Her blindness as to who Leonard really was may have been necessary for her to pursue her purpose. Her narrative was littered with clues alluding to how poorly Leonard had treated her and how worshipful she was towards him. Yet no she reflected no resentment in the way she spoke about him.

As for Leonard, it appeared that he didn't want to be married, but he *did* want to be financially supported, so that he could focus on nothing but his art and himself. He did not allow the marriage to interfere with or change his lifestyle in any way. Rachel's role was more breadwinner and housekeeper than significant other.

If the gap between Rachel's words and her understanding of their implications is removed, what of Rachel herself would be left? How much of that distance can be removed, and how much must remain?

Following Leonard's suicide, Rachel stayed "in character" as the inferior spouse whose life revolved around him, even though she no longer benefitted from the reflected glory of being married to a "great artist." She had been trying very hard to move on with her life, through every means available to her. She had seen psychologists and social workers, tried New Age treatments of various kinds, but nothing worked for her.

I asked Rachel to describe her home to me. She began by mentioning that Leonard's photographs still covered the walls. This despite the fact that for 12 years now, this was no longer *their* home, but *hers.*

I asked her, "Why?"

"To honor him."

"Why?" I reiterated. "He never honored you or treated you with respect. He was cruel to you. He was a waste of oxygen."

Her eyes widened in shock at my hard words. I thought perhaps I was too harsh. I asked her to continue describing her home.

"It's a small house. I have a living room, a dining room, a single bedroom, a kitchen, and two bathrooms, one for guests."

"Where are Leonard's photographs?"

"All over the walls of the living room, dining room, and kitchen."

In my past work, I had learned that the spouses of artists commonly live in their shadows. Whether or not this works for them when the artist is alive, the reflected glory is gone once the artist dies. However, the remaining artwork ensures the artist's continued dominance over the survivor's life.

"I imagine you feel better in the bathrooms and bedroom."

She pondered for a moment. "I do!" she suddenly responded, sounding surprised.

I waited for a moment to let her absorb the implication. Then I suggested a practical step to make her living space her own.

"You can't move on while he is still plastered all over your home, taking all the oxygen out of the air. Take all of his photographs off the walls. Take out the nails that held them. Fix any holes and cracks on the walls, and repaint the interior of the house."

Once the griever starts moving forward, even a little, it lends them strength for other, more emotionally demanding tasks.

"After that, call Leonard's son from his first marriage, and give all the photographs to him. Then, go shopping and look for something for your walls that gives you pleasure and allows you to breathe. Your house is not a mausoleum to be kept in his honor. The contract you two had—'until death parts us'—is over."

Rachel stared at me for a moment. Then she nodded in agreement. Now it was time to introduce *The Five Things* exercise.

"Next, write Leonard a letter. Before you sit down to write, make sure you are alone and cannot be disturbed. Turn off your phone. Prepare a writing space with something to drink, some tissues, a few pens, and a stack of paper. Go to the bathroom before you sit down to write."

"This letter is not meant to be a literary work; it's more like vomiting onto the page. Make no corrections, no crossing out, no erasing, and no rewrites. Begin the letter with: 'Leonard, it has been 12 years since we last spoke, and I have a few things I would like to say to you.' Then write whatever comes to your mind. It can be as long as you want. But write for at least 20 minutes. Do your best to make everything truthful and honest."

I continued: "There are five things that should be included in this letter:

1. 'Forgive me.'

Ask forgiveness for anything you did during your time together that you think may have hurt him in any way. And ask forgiveness for anything that, because you neglected to do it, may have hurt him. This has nothing to do with intent. You may apologize for any harm you inflicted on him, whether intentionally or unintentionally.

   2. 'I forgive you.'

Specifically include things that he did and said which hurt you, or things he didn't do and say that hurt you. Again, the intent, or lack thereof, is irrelevant.

   3. 'I loved you.'

You can specify why, when, how, or what it was you loved about him.

   4. 'Thank you.'

Mention the things for which you feel you should thank him. Do it honestly, be specific, and elaborate with specifics.

   5. 'Goodbye.'

This is last, a way of saying that it's over." [*]
"Make sure the letter is truthful and honest. After you write it, call me for an appointment. Bring the letter, because I will ask you to read it to me. If there is anything in it that you feel is too private to share, you can censor the reading, but you may *NOT* censor the writing."

"Can I ask a general kind of forgiveness?" she asked. "What if I apologize for all of the things at once?"

"Forgiveness is expensive," I explained. "You cannot ask for forgiveness from more than one person at a time. You cannot even ask forgiveness for more than one offense at a time. Forgiveness is a serious business. It is an exchange."

"And writing is a contract. It commits the writer to what they have written. Reading aloud is a declaration, and when it follows the writing, it has a freeing aspect to it."

Rachel called me a few days later, saying, "I want another appointment." We made one.

She arrived, looking like a different person. I barely recognized her. She was radiant.

"Talk to me," I urged her.

"Well, I took all the photographs down. There was a deep crack in the wall under one of the large ones. I called a handyman, and he took out all the nails, fixed and painted all the walls. The house seems so big, so light, so wonderful now."

[*]. See Recommended Reading no. 3.

"Then I called Leonard's son. He came over to pick up all of the photographs."

"Finally, I wrote the letter. But I want to know what I should do with our ketubah (traditional Jewish wedding contract) and my wedding ring."

"Let's put that question aside for a moment," I suggested, "while you read me the letter you wrote."

This is a way to buy time when the counselor doesn't have a ready answer. The issue might be clarified during the meeting, providing its own answer.

Rachel's letter was 24 pages long. It was a list of horrible things that were a part of her 6 years of marriage to a man who never really wanted to be married again, and who took it out on her.

She asked for his forgiveness for not being a wife he could be proud of, for never being bright enough for him. The list of what she forgave him for was detailed, including his unfaithfulness, his ridicule, his careless and sometimes intentional cruelty. She finished reading and looked at me calmly.

"When I wrote this, I was anything but calm. I cried and cried. But now it feels like it's over. . . . Resolved." She said the last word thoughtfully. Then she went on.

"When we first spoke about him, the man I loved and idealized, you shocked me to my core. I couldn't believe the things you were saying. Yet it was clear that they were true. I started writing as soon as I took the pictures off my walls. Once I got going, I could finally breathe. And so I kept on writing."

"What will you do with the letter?"

"I wanted to ask you what I should do."

"You could keep it . . ."

"I don't want to keep it."

". . . Or you could bury it. Or tie it to a helium balloon and let it fly away, or you could burn it . . ."

"Yes! That's what I'll do—I'll burn it!"

"Good," I replied. "That sounds good. What will you do with the ashes?"

"What can I do with the ashes?"

"You can put them on his grave."

"I know I should go to his grave, but it's hard. . . ."

"Then, don't go to his grave. You don't have to; it's finished."

"Maybe I can throw the ashes into the sea?"

"Sounds good. Now, what do you want to do with the ketubah?"

"I don't want it," she answered. "I'll give it to the rabbi."

"What about your wedding ring?"

This time, she didn't even hesitate. "I'll throw it into the sea, along with the ashes."

I sat back in admiration. "You are amazing, truly. I didn't think you could act on this so quickly. You are very strong."

I continued: "Now, I know you are feeling very good and powerful at the moment. But there will still be some tough times ahead. We have performed a kind of surgery, taking a lot of infection and debris out of your heart. Your heart is clean now, but the healing process will still cause some pain."

"However, you've also had a second surgery—you've had wings implanted on your back. They're still small and wet, but slowly they will grow, strengthen, and shine."

She just smiled.

NOTES TO THE PRACTITIONER

This case shows some of the complexities of grieving for a deceased abuser. First, we begin with the context. Leonard's photograph of his pregnant ex-wife in the home he shared with his current wife was cruel, in the context of Rachel's barrenness. In any case, displaying a photograph of a first wife is a slap in the second wife's face. So what would be the right intervention here?

Rachel provided all the information about her husband, but she was too emotionally involved to interpret that information. She was suffering from a blind spot that initially served her needs but cost her greatly in disappointment and guilt.

When Leonard married Rachel, she entered his world and left her own behind, because Leonard disapproved of her friends and acquaintances. She was isolated and entranced by what she was repeatedly told: he was a wonderful and amazing man. That left only herself to blame for whatever was going wrong between them. When she was suddenly presented with an external reflection of what she had lived with, she caught a glimpse of reality from a different angle.

As is usually the case after a suicide, Rachel was wracked with guilt about Leonard's death. His relatives, perhaps to abate their own feelings of guilt, pushed all of it onto her. Believing that she was to blame, and being in the throes of her own grief, Rachel accepted this guilt in a 12-year-long punishment.

The counselor needed to listen carefully to her stories, reorder her memories into a consolidated, meaningful whole, and reflect them back to her. Then, using practical tools, it was time to advise her on how to reclaim her home and life for herself.

Time does NOT heal all wounds. Wounds very often need help to heal. Or you have to find the little piece of torn soul stuck in the wound that is keeping the wound open and still running. . . . Find that, remove it, and clean the wound some; and it is amazing how fast it heals. (Eric Cassell, MD, personal correspondence)

CONCLUSIONS

- *To grieve a deceased abuser, it is necessary both to recognize the abuse and to forgive the abuser. This process in no way involves condoning or justifying the abuse.*
- *Meetings in the home are beneficial due to the information they offer. If this is not possible, asking for a description of the patient's home can also be revealing, both to counselors and counselees.*
- *Displayed objects, photographs or art, whether created by or given by the deceased, can make it difficult to continue living in the same place that the deceased once occupied.*
- *Practical tasks that can be completed quickly, whether large or small, can set the griever on the road to processing his or her grief.*

RECOMMENDED READING

1. Sarah LeTrent, "Death of an Unloved One," CNN (September 24, 2013), https:// edition.cnn.com/2013/09/24/living/death-anger-reddick-obit/index.html (accessed August 4, 2021).
2. Jo Baker, "When Abusive Relationships End: A Complex Grief," *Women's Counselling* (March 1, 2018), https://www.counselling-directory.org.uk/mem berarticles/when-abusive-relationships-end-a-complex-grief (accessed August 4, 2021).
3. "However, when I wrote out for him what hospice calls 'the five things of re-lationship completion'—saying 'I forgive you'; 'Forgive me'; 'Thank you'; 'I love you'; and 'Goodbye'—it gave him a kind of script with which to greet his final days with courage and determination." From Ira Byock, *Dying Well* (New York: Penguin Putnam, 1998), 139.

VI

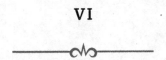

Communication-Related Concerns

20

∽

Quicksand

The Trap in Your Past

L indy's story is best told in her own words, without interruption:
   I am the second of five siblings. I was 14 years old, in junior high and living at home with my parents, when my grandfather came to live with us. He was a taciturn 93-year-old.

One morning, my mother told me: "You have a short school day, so when you come home, please give Grampa his lunch. It's in the fridge, on the second shelf. I will be out for most of the day."

When I came home from school, I remember dropping my books on the dining room table and taking off my boots.

Suddenly, I heard my grandfather's voice calling: "Help! Help me! Help . . ."

I ran towards the voice and saw that he was in the bathroom, with the door cracked open a little bit. He was sitting on the toilet, crying and pleading for help. I pushed the door open.

The entire bathroom was covered in feces: everywhere, on the walls, the floor, all over Grampa, on the little rug at his feet, his hands, his arms, and his legs. He was wailing and repeating, "I'm so ashamed, I'm so ashamed!"

I felt hollow. I looked around for a moment, and then I said, "It's okay, Grampa."

He kept on crying.

Clearing the Path. Lynne Dale Halamish and Eric J. Cassell, Oxford University Press. © Lynne Dale Halamish 2022.
DOI: 10.1093/oso/9780197636879.003.0020

I pulled him up from the toilet, his pants puddled around his ankles and his skinny white legs streaked with feces. I sat him back down again, knelt at his feet, and took off his shoes and socks. "It's okay, Grampa."

"I'm so ashamed," he muttered.

I slowly peeled his soiled pants and underwear off his legs, carefully removed his sweater, shirt, and undershirt, and dropped them to the floor.

It was the first time I had ever seen an adult male naked . . . 93 years old . . . his body covered in his own feces.

I walked him the few steps from the toilet to the bathtub and helped him step into it. I turned on the water, checked the temperature, and began to shower my Grampa. He stood helpless and crying in shame, and didn't lift a hand to help.

I finally rinsed and toweled him dry, then helped him out of the tub. Holding his arm firmly over my shoulder for support, I walked him through the mess to his bedroom, dressed him, and sat him down. I lit his pipe and handed it to him; he was weeping a bit less now. Then, I set up a folding table and got his lunch and a hot cup of tea. "It's okay, Grampa. Just eat a little. . . . Here, have some tea."

Once he was settled, I went back to the nightmare in the bathroom. My younger siblings would be home soon. I gathered up all the soiled clothes and brought them down to the basement, where I rinsed them in the big sink and shoved them into the washing machine. I added the proper amount of detergent, then added more, and turned on the wash.

After that, I went back to the bathroom with a bottle of bleach and began scrubbing the walls, the floors, the sink, and the bathtub.

Just as I was finishing up, I heard the younger sibs come into the house. I went out for a minute to remind them to take off their boots; they went on through the kitchen and got their lunch.

Two hours later, my mother walked in the door. I immediately started crying and couldn't speak. I started running up the stairs to my bedroom, and she raced after me to see what was wrong.

I cried and cried. My mother, not understanding, tried to comfort me, but to no avail. Then she went to see how Grampa and the other kids were doing. She returned with hot chocolate. By then, I had calmed down a bit, but tears were still streaming down my face.

"What happened?" my mother asked again.

"Grampa . . ." My voice cracked as I opened up. "He pooped all over himself and the bathroom. I . . . I had to clean it. And clean him, too. He . . . he was crying the whole time."

My mom held me tightly in silence for several minutes. When she let go, I could see that she had been crying also.

"I can't go downstairs," I told her desperately.

"It's all right, Lindy. Go take a bath, and I'll get you something to eat."

I didn't go to school the next day, or the day after that. I just stayed in my room, and I had all my meals in there, alone.

Now it's two and a half decades later, and here I am, a mother of four, caring for my elderly mother. She's dying from intestinal cancer. She had her right breast removed years ago, due to breast cancer. Now, she has a stoma and a bag attached to her body to collect her feces.

I've worked in nursing homes, and I've frequently bathed the sick and the elderly. So, it was reasonable when my mother called me over to her bed and asked, "Lindy, would you bathe me?"

I looked at her . . . and suddenly I was 14 years old again, standing in that feces-covered bathroom with my naked, crying grandfather.

"I . . . I can't," I answered her. But then the guilt washed over me. "Sorry, of course I will." Then I was back in the bathroom with Grampa again. "No . . . I just can't."

"But . . ." my mom said with surprise, "but, you've bathed lots of sick and elderly people."

I shook my head mutely. I couldn't even tell her why I couldn't do it. She would be horrified to hear that I somehow equated bathing her with that horrible, messy, shameful trauma.

How would *you* have advised Lindy?

NOTES TO THE PRACTITIONER

Sometimes as caretakers, whether professionals in the medical or psychosocial fields, or family members caring for loved ones, we feel we should be able to meet the patient's every need, particularly when they are dying.

So, what happens when we can't? Perhaps it's because we lack the physical or financial resources to answer every request. Maybe we don't have the *emotional* resources—which can happen for many reasons, including buried past trauma.

Are we allowed to say "no"?

Personally, I think not only are we allowed, but we *must*. We need to understand that no one can answer someone else's every need, no matter how much we wish we could, and it's best if we understand our limits in advance.

As I am sure some of you have already surmised, this is not a story about a client; it is part of my own story. I had "forgotten" that trauma for over two decades, until my dying mother asked me to bathe her. And I *could not do it*. Nor could I bring myself to tell her why.

Nevertheless, it is interesting to ponder how such painful experiences can shape our lives.

A few months after the adventure—or misadventure—with my grandfather, I began visiting nursing homes and retirement communities (still a 14-year-old), just to look at the people there. Then, I began to sketch pictures of the desperately poor elderly. Later, I volunteered in retirement homes and geriatric hospital departments. By the time I went off to university, my choice to major in Gerontology and then Thanatology was hardly a big surprise.

I don't know whether that day as a young girl with my grandfather was indeed the first step towards my career as a thanatologist, but it was unquestionably one of them.

CONCLUSIONS

- *Try to identify in advance your own vulnerable points that might limit you in answering requests from the dying for certain kinds of care.*
- *If you stumble across a vulnerability by surprise, note it and prepare for the next time; if necessary, refer the patient to someone who is better equipped to help them.*
- *You are not doing the patient or loved one any favors when you take on a task that you are clearly unable to do.*
- *If your gut reaction has proven reliable in the past, trust it. At the very least, do not ignore it.*

RECOMMENDED READING

1. "Caring for Someone Nearing the End of Life," *Cancer Council Victoria*, https://www.cancervic.org.au/get-support/facing-end-of-life/caring-for-someone-nearing-the-end-of-life (accessed August 4, 2021).
2. "Coping with Feelings as a Carer," *Marie Curie* (February 5, 2021), https://www.mariecurie.org.uk/help/support/being-there/helping-someone-cope/dealing-with-feelings (accessed August 4, 2021).

21

∿

The Petrified Woman

Making Assumptions

I received a call from a woman named Marina one morning.

She explained, "We met about a year ago, at one of your lectures. I work with a woman named Sonya Seigel; you spoke with her briefly right after your lecture. She has asked me to arrange a meeting with you."

I definitely remembered that earlier meeting with Sonya, a woman who suffered from quadriplegia. Marina had been with her then also, and had told me that Sonya wanted a word with me following my lecture.

I came over to her massive, chin-activated wheelchair, sat down in a chair slightly below her eye level, and smiled. I asked her what it was she wanted to ask me. She answered in a kind of wheezing voice, taking a deep breath and then pushing it out in order to speak. The volume of her voice dropped with each syllable, until she ran completely out of breath. I couldn't catch it all, so Marina explained Sonya's question to me.

Now, Sonya was making an appointment with me. I was slightly nervous about how I could even help her when I couldn't understand what she was saying. I asked Marina why she wanted to meet.

"She's depressed," she told me.

How could she *not* be depressed? I thought. She couldn't move any of her limbs, could barely talk. And how could *I* help her, when her state of utter helplessness was horrifying to me?

I suggested that perhaps a psychologist would be a better option for her. No, Marina insisted, Sonya only wanted to meet with me.

Clearing the Path. Lynne Dale Halamish and Eric J. Cassell, Oxford University Press. © Lynne Dale Halamish 2022.
DOI: 10.1093/oso/9780197636879.003.0021

I went to the home of Sonya's friends, where she spent some of her afternoons and weekends. This was an alternative that allowed her to get away from the assisted-living housing where she usually lived. We met in a lovely garden. It was a mild, balmy day, and the cool breeze was lightly rustling the leaves all around us.

Sonya was a small woman of about 40. She was obviously well cared for, wearing a lovely outfit, mascara, and lipstick. Her long hair was neatly brushed and pinned back with a pearl barrette. She smiled as I approached her. I sat in the chair that had been placed near her.

"Hello, Sonya. I understand that you wanted to see me?"

Sonya began her wheezing speech. I leaned forward to try and make out her words through her raspy breaths. Little by little, I began to make out the words. I couldn't catch everything at first, but slowly, using a great deal of concentration, I began to understand her.

I asked Sonya to tell me how she lost the use of her limbs. She related the story slowly:

"At the age of 13, I immigrated with my parents and brother from Romania. I was born with one leg somewhat shorter than the other, causing me to limp. When my family was finally settled, we found a family physician who was convinced that it could be fixed with surgery."

While she was speaking, a fly landed on her left cheek. She couldn't brush it off. She couldn't even shake her head to make it go away. Coming face to face with her helplessness made me extremely uneasy. I didn't feel familiar enough with her to brush the fly away for her.

She continued her narrative: "An operation was scheduled to fix my slightly shorter left leg. But I came out of the operating room laterally paralyzed on my entire left side. My left arm and leg simply stopped working. The surgeon said he could fix it, so of course, I went under the knife again. Not only was he unable to restore my left side, but my entire right side became paralyzed, too, making me quadriplegic."

So, it was the result of an iatrogenic injury . . . in plain language, a medical mistake. My nervousness grew as I anticipated dealing with her depression. I asked her if she could move her limbs at all. She smiled and said, "Yes, of course I can."

I asked her to show me. She made a tiny, incremental movement with her right hand—sort of a slight shake.

A refreshing breeze came through the garden, and one of Sonya's long hairs was swept up and over her face, clinging to her lipstick. I stared at it uncomfortably, knowing that she couldn't move it.

I asked how she managed her personal care, how she was dressed so well, how she used the telephone or brushed her teeth, and more.

She told me of the care she received from her caregivers. Many were good, particularly those she was able to hire when her budget would allow it. In the assisted-living institution, they were less good. Sometimes caregivers were even physically abusive to her while "caring" for her body. But she seemed to regard this as normal and not particularly distressing.

She also told me that she chose all her own clothing, and that she liked some brands and colors more than others. She shared her desire to get her own apartment someday. She even had a boyfriend at the institution, who always sat next to her and would constantly tell her how beautiful and smart she is. She smiled when she spoke of him.

She said that she was blessed by a benevolent God. She had a place of worship she attended where she prayed regularly, and she felt loved by many there.

"And I'm an artist!" she announced with a sparkle in her eye.

"An artist?" I was unable to mask my astonishment.

"Yes, I am a mouth painter. Someone dips the brush for me in the color I want, places it in my mouth, and I paint. I would love to have an exhibition."

I was bewildered by her upbeat attitude. I could not see any signs of depression, much less understand how I could help with it.

Finally, I had to ask point-blank. "Sonya, why did you want to meet with me today?"

Suddenly Sonya's face fell, her luminous smile fading away. "My brother died a week ago. I want you to help me with my grief."

I was startled at the basic mistake I had made.

I had been assuming that I knew what Sonya needed, before she actually told me. And having assumed, I had concluded that I had no tools that could possibly help a depression born of such helplessness. Neither idea had anything to do with the person sitting before me.

Sonya didn't feel helpless. She had dreams that she believed would one day come true. She had a strong faith in a benevolent God. She felt beautiful and loved. She was a passionate artist.

And just like everyone else whom I had been privileged to serve, she was struggling with a normal, familiar problem: grief over the loss of a beloved brother.

I think I learned more during that one meeting with Sonya than she did.

NOTES TO THE PRACTITIONER

When it comes to the human experience, there is no guarantee of a shared response to reality. Each response depends on how that person views the situation through his or her own experiential lens. This was made very clear in my encounter with Sonya. Her physical limitations were challenging for me to watch, while she was coping admirably with them—and clearly had been doing so for some time.

A meeting between two people is a collision between two worlds. Sometimes they meet with a crash, and other times with a gentle nudge. We have to peer past our own biases and opinions to see the other person clearly. This involves attentive listening and awareness of body language, in order to discover what the client or patient is really telling us.

The experience of actively listening allows us to be less biased; it removes assumptions. This provides a strong healing process both for the patient and his family, and it is also a gratifying experience for us as professionals. If we experience gratification in our work, we care for our patients and their families much better, and we experience less burnout. (Y. Singer, MD, personal correspondence)

When we jump to conclusions, as I initially did, we risk missing the main issue. Instead of making assumptions, ask detailed questions until you know, beyond a doubt, that you are seeing and hearing the person in front of you.

CONCLUSIONS

- *Do not make assumptions. You do not know anything for sure, unless you ask.*
- *Be aware of your own fears, and the risk of projecting them onto the people you serve.*

RECOMMENDED READING

1. Heather S. Lonczak, "33 Counseling Mistakes Therapists Should Avoid and How to Prevent Them," *Positive Psychology* (January 9, 2020), https://positivepsychol ogy.com/things-therapists-should-not-do/ (accessed August 4, 2021).

2. "Research Reveals Why Humans Often Make Wrong Assumptions," *Power of Positivity* (August 14, 2020), https://www.powerofpositivity.com/assumptions-jumping-to-conclusions/ (accessed August 4, 2021).

22

⌘

The Silent Woman

Messages That Go Unheard

The two women who called me were in their mid-40s and wanted me to
speak with their mother. She was suffering from a terminal disease, but
that wasn't the whole problem.

"We really want you to come and talk to her, but she has become a horrible woman. She screams at anyone who comes into her room, swearing
like a drunken sailor. She tries to hit people who approach her. She has
gone so far as to spit in some of her caretakers' faces. She will not even let
us, her daughters, come close."

"Okay," I replied. "How about Wednesday at 10 am?"

"You don't understand how awful she is."

"Do you want me to come and meet with your mother?"

"Yes, but . . ."

"Is Wednesday at 10 all right?"

"Yes. Please."

I arrived on schedule. I was still wiping my feet on the welcome mat
when the two daughters met me at the door, once again telling me how
positively dreadful their mother was.

My response was abrupt. "Look, I only have 1 hour. Would you like me
to go in and see her or not?"

"Yes, of course. Please be careful." Their apologetic voices were still following me as I made my way towards the bedroom door at the end of the
hallway.

Clearing the Path. Lynne Dale Halamish and Eric J. Cassell, Oxford University Press. © Lynne Dale Halamish 2022.
DOI: 10.1093/oso/9780197636879.003.0022

I entered a large, white-walled bedroom. Sunlight was pouring in from an expansive window, illuminating a small woman lying in a large bed with white sheets. I looked around and saw that a chair stood by the opposite wall; I silently walked over, picked it up, put it close to the bed, and sat down.

Neither of us had said a single word.

The woman's hands were clenched at her side as she eyed me with big, green, wary eyes. I held her gaze and waited in silence. After several minutes, the hand closest to me started to unclench and slowly turned over, palm up. The silent woman carefully watched me, slightly tilting her head in my direction. I waited a little longer and then gently placed my hand into hers. We both closed our hands, clasping the other's hand lightly, eyes still locked in a mute gaze.

My face was directly towards hers, and gradually her head tilted more and more towards me until we were looking at each other straight on. The silence was still unbroken.

But the communication was strong. I felt like I was being drawn into her eyes, making a connection with someone whom I hadn't known existed until now—but whom I suddenly cared for, deeply. It felt, strangely enough, like falling in love.

After about 20 minutes of looking deeply into each other's eyes without making a sound, she opened her hand, and I did likewise. I gently lifted my hand out of hers and stood up.

"Thank you," said the no-longer-silent woman.

I smiled and then I walked over to the door and opened it.

The woman's daughters fell tumbling into the room. They had apparently been leaning against the door, trying to hear.

They quickly regained their balance and gave a frightened glance at their mother, as they backed out through the open doorway. I turned and looked back at her with a small smile, which she echoed back at me. I then left the room, shutting the door behind me.

"So? What happened?" her daughters asked me breathlessly.

"We communicated," I replied.

"What did you say? What did *she* say?"

"Counselor–client privilege," I replied, and I left the house.

This encounter with the silent woman occupied my thoughts for the rest of that day. When my husband came home from work that evening, he asked, "How did it go with the 'scary woman' you were meeting with today?"

I smiled at the memory. "She wasn't horrible, just a small, sickly old woman. And if I'm not mistaken, I think I fell in love with her."

This was the first and last time I ever saw this woman. She died shortly afterwards. I am still not entirely sure what exactly happened that day, but I do know that there was a profound interchange between us in that silence.

NOTES TO THE PRACTITIONER

It's significant that since ancient times, the Hebrew expression for "pay attention" has always been literally to "put your heart" to it. This concept preserves the wisdom that real attention demands listening with one's heart.

Sometimes your patient or client will not communicate in the ways you expect. Nonverbal communication comprises between 85% and 93% of all human interaction. Pay close attention to the body language of the person you are trying to communicate with, and they will show you how to proceed. You will find indications that they are indeed "talking" to you beyond the words, or even without words.

Abraham Lincoln once observed, "The more a man speaks, the less he is understood." When faced with a breakdown in communication, silence can be a powerful tool.

This is a difficult and even counterintuitive response, but it's well worth the effort. As we saw in previous chapters, a silent, actively listening counselor provides a stage for the client to communicate without hindrance, while also reducing the accumulated "noise" (both from well-meaning comforters and from inside the mourner) which hampers clear communication.

CONCLUSIONS

- *Misinterpretations can create barriers in communication and make it even harder to understand one another; this in turn exacerbates the patient's sense of isolation.*
- *In nonverbal communication, the most powerful tool I have encountered is silence.*
- *Whether or not we use words, we can never absolutely ascertain what each of the parties understood from the interchange. Therefore, nonverbal communication can be as effective as words.*

RECOMMENDED READING

1. Kurt Smith, "Silence: The Secret Communication Tool," *PsychCentral* (October 6, 2014), https://psychcentral.com/blog/silence-the-secret-communication-tool#1 (accessed August 4, 2021).
2. "Usually, when we make a mistake, it is not because we are listening too much. In communication with the griever, there is never room for more than one on the stage. This means if you are talking, you are not listening. If you are really listening, you are not talking. You either take the stage or relinquish it to someone else." From L. Halamish and D. Hermoni, "The Silent Stage," in *The Weeping Willow: Encounters with Grief* (New York: Oxford University Press, 2007), 49.

VII

Other Topics and Concerns

Other Topics and Concerns

23

༄

The Cornerman

Defining Your Work

At age 39, David was a young widower. His wife had died suddenly in a car crash, leaving him alone with three children, aged 7, 10, and 14.

David had come to me 4 days after his wife's death, convinced that his life was over. He claimed that he would have "joined her" in death, were it not for his three children. He was convinced that he would never smile again, never love again. He was facing the biggest challenge of his life.

Throughout the time we met, I emphasized that all grief has a beginning, a middle, and a *possible* end (see Chapter 30, "Surviving Death: The End of Grief"). I assured him that he would not always feel the way he was feeling right now. Grief is a process, a dynamic path, not a place of residence.

Now, after a year of intervention, we were meeting for the last time. David had come a long way over the past year. He had changed jobs, learned how to run his household on his own, redefined himself, taken help where he needed it. He had even—to his immense surprise—found a new love.

He was very grateful for the time we spent together. "I could never have done any of this without you. You did it all," he said to me.

"No, no, David," I responded. "Let me explain what my part was in your uphill climb: I was in your corner."

"Exactly!" he answered. "You fought this fight for me."

"No, this was *your* fight. But I am in your corner." He stared at me, perplexed. So I explained what that expression actually means.

Clearing the Path. Lynne Dale Halamish and Eric J. Cassell, Oxford University Press. © Lynne Dale Halamish 2022.
DOI: 10.1093/oso/9780197636879.003.0023

"As a youth, my father was a boxer," I began. "So, in my childhood home, we used a lot of boxing slang. As you know, the game is held in a square called a ring. The boxers go into the middle for 3-minute rounds, with a 1-minute interval between them. When the bell rings at the end of the round, each boxer goes back to his corner of the ring. The cornermen, or trainers, or 'cut men,' as they are variously called, provide assistance and advice to the boxer. The cornerman places a folding chair in the corner for the boxer to sit on, takes out his mouthpiece, gives him water and advice, wipes down his face."

I continued: "And if, for example, the boxer has taken a punch to the eye, and it's swollen shut, the cornerman slices the eyelid open, pushes out the fluids, and tapes the skin high, so the boxer can see. Then, the cornerman advises him on strategy for the next round and sends the boxer back out into the fight."

"*That's* my job. I'm your cornerman, while *you* are the one in the ring taking and giving the punches. Everything that was achieved, you have done. The fight is yours to win or lose; I'm just doing my best to make sure you make it back in, to fight another round."

NOTES TO THE PRACTITIONER

As flattering as receiving the credit can be, it is not helpful to the patient or counselee to think that they need someone else to achieve their goals for them. Our objective, particularly in counseling, is to empower, not to encourage dependence. The building-up process must be honest, but take note of your patient's every achievement and acknowledge each one verbally, to strengthen and encourage them.

As physicians, sometimes our expertise can be what has saved the patient, and that recognition can be accepted. But the arduous journey back to health is primarily dependent on adherence to directions, physiotherapy, and pharmacological regimens. These are all, ultimately, in the hands of the patient.

CONCLUSIONS

- *Don't take credit, even in your own mind, for transformative changes in your patients.*
- *Acknowledge patients' bravery, temerity, or constancy, or whatever it took for them to make the changes or the decisions that helped them. The merit belongs to the patients.*

> • *We are a source of medical or other assistance, support, and information. The patient is on the front line.*

RECOMMENDED READING

1. Rebecca J. Frey, "Bereavement Counseling," Encyclopedia.com (updated December 25, 2020), https://www.encyclopedia.com/caregiving/encyclopedias-almanacs-transcripts-and-maps/bereavement-counseling (accessed August 4, 2021).
2. Kurt C. Stange, "Identifying Personal Strengths to Help Patients Manage Chronic Illness," Case Western Reserve University research project (September 21, 2020), https://www.pcori.org/research-results/2012/identifying-personal-strengths-help-patients-manage-chronic-illness (accessed August 4, 2021).

24

⌁

The Ripple Effect

Who Will Leave Next?

When Nathaniel was born, he had a lot of elderly relatives. Besides the four usual grandparents (his parents' parents), he also had four great-grandparents, for a rare total of eight living grandparents!

To a small child in the family-oriented culture of Israel, this seemed like a great advantage. And for a short while, it was. But by the time he turned 6, Nathaniel had lost two great-grandparents and another two of his grandparents.

One of his remaining grandmothers, Gayle, was preparing him to attend the funeral for the most recently deceased grandmother. It would be Nathaniel's first time attending a burial.

She asked the boy, as they sat side by side on the yard swing below the old willow tree, "Do you remember that Grandma Dinah died?"

"Yes," Nathaniel answered, staring at his knees as he kicked his legs back and forth, back and forth, rocking the swing lightly under himself and his Gramma Gayle.

"Do you remember why she died?"

"Yes," his little face suddenly looked up and met her eyes. "Cancer."

"What is cancer?" Gramma Gayle asked.

"A sickness."

"How does someone get cancer?"

"A crab bites you on the beach," he replied.

Clearing the Path. Lynne Dale Halamish and Eric J. Cassell, Oxford University Press. © Lynne Dale Halamish 2022.
DOI: 10.1093/oso/9780197636879.003.0024

This was childlike logic. In Hebrew, the word for *cancer* refers to the disease, the zodiac sign, and the sea animal.

"No," said Gayle, and she paused until little Nathaniel raised his eyes again. "It's not from a crab. We don't really know why she got it."

He wrinkled his forehead. "She smoked cigarettes."

"That may be why, but we're not sure that was the cause."

"You don't know *everything*, Gramma."

"That's right, I don't know *everything*. But I do know this."

Their conversation had to halt for a few moments, as a hummingbird hovered for a few moments a few feet away, which prompted Nathaniel to whisper excitedly so as not to scare it away. After it flew off and he settled down again, Gramma Gayle continued with what she "did know."

"Now we have to do something with Grandma Dinah's body."

"Her body goes to heaven," Nathaniel replied confidently.

"No, she doesn't need her body anymore." Nathaniel's eyes widened at the new idea. "It was sick, it was a mess. Her *spirit* goes to heaven."

"Oh! So . . . What should we do with the body?" he asked her.

"What *should* we do?" she asked him.

"I don't know, Gramma Gayle." He shrugged.

"Well, in our family culture, we take her body and clean it. Then, we put a new clean cloth on it, called a shroud." She paused. Nathaniel's eyes were fixed on hers.

"Then we take her body to where we put the bodies of people who die. This is called a graveyard. In the graveyard, there is a hole in the ground that has been dug for Grandma Dinah, and we will put her body there because she no longer needs it."

She paused again, looking carefully at Nathaniel. He was still paying attention, sitting in silence.

"Then," she went on, "we cover the body up with earth. Later, we put a stone there with her name on it, to remember where her body is. Then, if we feel like we miss her, and we want to, we can go there."

They continued to sit together quietly for a while.

"Tell me something, Nathaniel. Does Grandma Dinah need food to eat now?"

"No."

"Right. She doesn't need food, because she died. Is she cold?"

"No."

"Right, because she is no longer alive. Can anything happen to her body that will hurt her?"

"No."

"Right, because she isn't there in her body anymore."

That afternoon, Nathaniel attended the funeral in his father's arms, with his grandmother by his side. He carefully observed the proceedings and asked a few questions.

Some days later, he was sitting with his grandmother on the porch swing again. Nathaniel's little hand was holding a drippy ice cream cone.

"Gramma Gayle?" He looked at her.

"Yes, Nathaniel?"

"Never mind." He quickly looked down at his ice cream.

"What is it, Nathaniel?"

"Nothing."

"Nathaniel, do you have a question?" Gramma Gayle looked into his eyes.

"Yes . . . No. I don't."

"You can ask me anything, Nathaniel; it doesn't matter what the question is."

"Um," he stared at his hands holding the cone, and his voice became softer as he whispered, "Gramma Gayle, are you going to die, too?"

Gayle looked at her oldest grandson tenderly. "I will, eventually. But I don't think it will happen soon; you will probably be all grown up by the time I die."

"What if you get sick? Like Grandma Dinah?" he asked with a small voice.

"Don't worry, Nathaniel. If I get sick, I will let you know."

Nathaniel sighed in relief. There was no immediate threat, and he was able to voice his fears.

"Gramma, what's a 'spirit'?"

"A spirit?" To gain time, Gayle removed her glasses and wiped them with the edge of her shirt.

"You said Grandma Dinah's spirit goes to heaven."

"Ahh. What do *you* think a spirit is, Nathaniel?"

"Um . . . A ghost?" He whispered.

"No, not a ghost," Gramma Gayle smiled. The spirit is from God, it's like a part of Him, so it can never die. It's Grandma Dinah's, but it also belongs to God."

"Oh! Then *I* know what it is!" The child's eyes suddenly sparkled as he jumped up from the swing, momentarily startling his grandmother.

"Really? Would you mind explaining to me?"

"The spirit is not God, but it's the part of God that He gives to us so it can't die."

"Ok . . . And what part of God do you think that is?"

"Grandma—don't you know? It's God's love."

NOTES TO THE PRACTITIONER

Children often get pushed to the sidelines when it comes to a death in the family. This is usually done with good intentions, trying to shield the child from the pain of grief. However, instead of protecting, it does the child a disservice. It can alienate children from their support system, which is usually the immediate or extended family.

A more effective protection for the child is inclusion, not only in times of joy but also in times of family difficulty, pain, and sorrow. We need to give them their rightful place in the grievers' circle so that they, too, can be comforted. Children, with their simple perceptions, can also be an unexpected source of comfort to the adults as well. Or at least a periodic distraction from grief during the mourning period.

With most children, the most effective way to do this is to give them attention, and a stage to express themselves by asking them simple, direct questions. Give them due credit for their answers, and correct any misconceptions they might have relating to the subject.

All counseling of children should respect both the age-appropriate framework of explanation and the acceptable norms of the child's family and culture. Everything that the child expresses as his or her ideas or personal beliefs should be honored, just as we would hopefully do with an adult, and just as we expect our ideas to be honored by others.

In this clinical tale, it is evident that if Nathaniel had not been pressed to reveal one of his questions, he would have been nervous and fearful about losing another grandparent, and no one would have known to address it. This fear is superfluous and can be attended to with minimal effort by an honest conversation, as illustrated here, at ages as young as 6 and even earlier.

CONCLUSIONS

- *Children are entitled to participate in family events, whether joyful or otherwise.*
- *When children are not permitted to participate in family events, they become sidelined and isolated.*
- *If their questions are not addressed, superfluous or unnecessary fears may take root.*

RECOMMENDED READING

1. Anya Kamenetz and Cory Turner, "Be Honest and Concrete: Tips for Talking to Kids about Death," *NPR Parenting: Difficult Conversations* (May 28, 2020), https://www.npr.org/2019/04/24/716702066/death-talking-with-kids-about-the-end (accessed August 4, 2021).
2. Deborah Serani, "The Do's and Don'ts of Talking with a Child about Death," *Psychology Today* (December 4, 2016), https://www.psychologytoday.com/us/blog/two-takes-depression/201612/the-dos-and-donts-talking-child-about-death (accessed August 4, 2021).

25

cⁿ⌀

Senicide

Suicide Contagion

I was meeting with 85-year-old Amelia in the nursing home where she resided. I had been asked to come and meet with her by the staff social worker, who claimed that Amelia had been depressed recently.

"You know," Amelia remarked to me, "my son's mother-in-law was a woman of very high standards and ethics."

"Really?" I waited to hear why this third person was relevant to our conversation.

"Yes, she was," replied Amelia firmly. "She was also courageous. Everyone says so."

"Hmmm." I said noncommittally and continued to look at her. I observed that instead of returning my gaze, she looked slightly to the side. She continued to explain.

"Three years ago—she was 78, suffering from a chronic disease—she was supposed to come into this nursing home where I now live. Instead, she got into a golf cart and went to the local swimming pool after hours. She went right up to the edge of the pool, drove herself with her golf cart into the water, and drowned. She was fearless, and everyone was amazed by her courage. It makes me feel like . . ."

She looked at me and paused for a moment. "Perhaps . . . I should be that courageous."

I continued to look at her silently.

Amelia pushed me for a response. "Don't *you* think she was brave?"

Clearing the Path. Lynne Dale Halamish and Eric J. Cassell, Oxford University Press. © Lynne Dale Halamish 2022.
DOI: 10.1093/oso/9780197636879.003.0025

I gathered my thoughts and replied. "She may have had many ethical and moral standards, but she didn't have enough of them."

"What?" Amelia tilted her head as if she thought she had misheard me.

"She may have endangered the lives of her whole family by willfully ending her life."

Amelia was now confused. "I don't understand."

"Once you open this door, this option to end your own life, it stays open. . . . It becomes an option for your children, grandchildren, great-grandchildren, friends, siblings, and anyone else who has ever known you."

Amelia remained silent but very attentive. I continued.

"At the time, you feel that you are suffering. Well, a child who fails a math test may also feel he is suffering. Teenagers who have a bad complexion may feel they are suffering. The kids who are humiliated or bullied on social media may feel they have no more reason to live. And if you have modeled suicide as a solution for suffering, it's an option also for the child."

"This is actually known to be infectious. It's called 'suicide contagion.' You want to know how infectious it is? Your son's mother-in-law did this 3 years ago, and even though you aren't her blood relative, you're influenced enough by it to consider emulating her."

We sat in silence for a few minutes.

"You know," said Amelia thoughtfully, "I had another friend who was not completely healthy but not disabled in any way, and yet she killed herself, too. She was in her mid-60s. She wrote letters to everyone— her family, friends, and even sent a letter to be published in the newspaper that day. She wrote a whole essay about how she didn't want to be a drain on the community's resources. She suggested in her public letter that everyone over 70 should follow her example. This was about 16 years ago."

"How did the community respond?" I asked.

"Everyone was furious with her! Her husband was somewhat crippled and needed her care, and she just left him. She left everyone behind. People felt it was unjustified and selfish and were outraged. Particularly because she said that everyone should do the same."

Amelia paused, pondering. "But still . . . I heard that many secretly tried to find out how she did it, and where she got such a detailed plan. . . . Some of them quietly talked about doing the same someday."

I remembered that newspaper article. I had also heard that response.

"You said, as I remember, that you don't believe in God?" I inquired.

"No. I don't."

"And you don't believe that there is anything after death?"

"No."

"In that case, what's your hurry? You have nowhere better to go. According to what you say, there's nowhere at all to go." I paused. "This step is irreversible."

"I am so tired, though." Her eyes seemed to be filling with tears. She lifted her chin, slightly shaking her head swiftly from side to side, as if she just didn't know what to do.

I appealed to reason. "You're taking strong antibiotics. You'll be done in a week. Perhaps a week or two after that, you'll feel stronger. Maybe. Maybe not. But nonetheless, you are a mother."

"Yes."

"You are a grandmother."

"Yes."

"And you are, I think, a great-grandmother also?"

"Yes, I am." She grinned proudly. "Of four, no less!"

"Your responsibility, as a mother, is to protect your children. If you kill yourself, or act to end your life in any way, you could be endangering your children and your children's children. You have *no right* to do this. Things are hard. But you are already . . . what? Eighty-five years old? And not very healthy?"

"That's right."

"How much time do you have left to suffer—till 120?!" I was referring to the traditional birthday greeting in Israel: "May you live to 120," the age of Moses when he died.

She looked startled for a moment, and we both burst out laughing.

Humor is a valuable therapeutic tool, and it can be used very effectively—as long as we ensure that all understand that we are not laughing *at* the patient and family, but *with* them.

As I was leaving 15 minutes later, Amelia grasped my hand in both of hers and smiled like the sun coming out. "Thank you. Thank you so much," she said.

I returned to Amelia the following week. She seemed happier, more vibrant; she reported feeling more contented with life. "What changed?" I asked her.

She smiled that sunny smile. "I needed a good shaking, and you gave it to me! I wanted to be remembered as 'brave,' to have people talk about me the way they talk about those others. I felt as though I should relieve my family of my existence by ending it . . . so as not to be selfish. You gave me a reason not to feel like a burden."

She paused, considering. "Instead, you reminded me of my parental role. Protecting my children and their children. You gave me a new perspective and condemned suicide in a way I had never heard before."

Later that same week, I met with Amelia's family: her husband and three adult children. We spoke about Amelia, who she was to them, and who they were to her. I also shared with them how actively ending a life, even at an advanced age like Amelia's, may endanger the survivors.

I explained, "We cannot decide to end our life when something is unbearable. Children and youth are especially dramatic. What would be a minor event to us can cause great anguish for a child or teen, who might also decide that life is unbearable."

They were visibly shaken at the implications of what I was saying.

"This is not a new discovery or a unique effect," I explained further. "In a family where divorce has occurred, divorce among the grown children is more likely. Where alcoholism exists, drinking as an escape becomes more legitimate. Battered children often grow up to be battering parents. And in this case, we are talking about life and death. No take-backs, no second chances."

I continued, watching them carefully. "Perhaps you have even admired or praised sick or elderly people who committed suicide to supposedly relieve their families of an unwanted burden. Perhaps Amelia even heard you when you did."

They looked at each other guiltily and admitted that they had responded that way. I then came to the point as gently as possible.

"Your mother is in an excellent nursing home in your community and receives outstanding care. She is happy and safe there, and she has a private room where you can all come and visit. She is lucid, lovely, and witty. But . . ." I paused for emphasis, "even she felt almost an obligation to kill herself because it was admired and—in a way—expected."

NOTES TO THE PRACTITIONER

This is primarily a clinical tale about peer pressure, or social and familial pressure. It is also about paying attention to whom you are speaking, and who can hear your voice. This is especially important for health practitioners in hallway conversations.

This is likewise a story that identifies suicide, regardless of the motivation, as possibly dangerous to the surroundings of the one who commits the act. We know very well that all actions have consequences, repercussions, and side effects. With this in mind, is "not being a burden" an adequate reason to end a life?

In current society, the traditional role of the elderly in passing on acquired wisdom has been reduced, if not erased, by the accessibility of online information. So, what role do they still hold? One passive role of the elderly is to serve as an example.

On a functional level, which role of the elderly remains they are keepers of their family history. They also have the knowledge accumulated in life experience, although that seems to be valued less today as well.

Out of the Ten Commandments, only one comes with a reward: "Honor your father and mother, that your days may be prolonged in the land which the Lord your God gives you" (Exodus 20:12). What this means, on a practical level, is that your children are watching the way you treat your parents and will someday feel justified in treating you the same way.

Lastly, there is a moral debt involved. Your parents raised you? There is a debt to be paid to them.

CONCLUSIONS

- *Pay attention to the relational dynamics influencing your patient, especially suicide contagion.*
- *When considering an action—any action—try to think of the possible repercussions.*
- *Sometimes when we prescribe medication, the side effects are worse than the disease it is treating. This also applies to communication.*

RECOMMENDED READING

1. This article discusses factors that increase the risk of suicide contagion when reporting a suicide. It proposes focusing on warning signs and prevention resources in news coverage to reduce that risk. Sima Patel, "Suicide Contagion: What We Know and What We Don't," *ABC News* (June 8, 2018), https://abcnews.go.com/Health/suicide-contagion/story?id=55751220 (accessed August 5, 2021).
2. This article reviews evidence that supports the concept of suicide contagion in three bodies of research (Jacobson and Gould 2009; Hawton et al. 2010; Whitlock 2010). It then focuses specifically on attempted and completed suicide. Madelyn S. Gould and Alison M. Lake, "The Contagion of Suicidal Behavior," *NCBI Resources* (2013), ahttps://www.ncbi.nlm.nih.gov/books/NBK207262/ (accessed August 5, 2021).
3. Tori Rodriguez, "Expert Roundtable: A Close Look at Suicide 'Contagion,'" *Psychiatry Advisor* (June 6, 2019), https://www.psychiatryadvisor.com/home/topics/general-psychiatry/expert-roundtable-a-close-look-at-suicide-contagion/ (accessed August 5, 2021).

26

✧

The Threat

How Do You Know It's Real?

Harriet was 82 years old and recently widowed from her husband of 50 years. Yes, they had been married for half a century. Harriet met Eli when she was 30, and they married 2 years later. They raised four children together, who were now their mid-to-late 40s, and they had seven grandchildren.

"When did your husband die?" I asked her at our first meeting.

"Thirty-two days ago," she replied. "I thought I could manage by myself. I thought I was so strong, but now I am just so sad all the time. I no longer work much, and many of my friends have already died. The small apartment we shared seems so large and hollow without Eli."

"That must be very difficult," I said.

"Yes, it is. But I've made a decision."

"What is your decision?" I asked.

"I am going to join him." The wrinkles across her forehead deepened.

"What do you mean?"

"I will kill myself," she said plainly.

It was time to evaluate her seriousness. Was suicide an immediate threat? Did she have a viable plan?

"How?" I asked.

She responded immediately, "Pills."

"Do you have any?" I asked.

Clearing the Path. Lynne Dale Halamish and Eric J. Cassell, Oxford University Press. © Lynne Dale Halamish 2022.
DOI: 10.1093/oso/9780197636879.003.0026

She eyed me, stood up, and walked out of the room. I heard a bit of shuffling around, and she returned moments later, carrying a shoebox. She sat back down, eyed me again for a moment, and then lifted the lid. The box was filled almost to the brim with pills of every shape and color.

I raised my eyebrows. This amount of pills had obviously not been collected in the month that had passed since her husband died.

"When do you plan to kill yourself?" I asked.

"I haven't decided yet," said Harriet quietly.

"Before our meeting next week?"

"No, I don't think so," she replied.

After talking to her for about an hour, I made a final request regarding the suicide ideation. "Okay, so let's make a verbal contract, you and I, that if you change your mind, you must contact me. Contact me *before* you take action. Not leaving a message, either. You must reach me and speak with me. Do we have a deal?"

She looked at me carefully and extended her hand to shake mine. With a firm grip we shook hands, looking into each other's eyes intently. "Deal," she said.

This "verbal contract" carried a certain amount of risk, but despite Harriet having a plan and the means to carry it out, I assessed that she was no in immediate danger.

Sure enough, we kept on meeting for several months—considerably longer than my average counseling period. I started each meeting by asking Harriet a series of questions:

"Are you still planning to kill yourself?"

"Yes."

"With pills?"

"Yes."

"You have the pills?"

"Yes."

"Before next week?"

"No."

"Do you agree not to do it without contacting me first?"

"Yes."

Then we would continue our meeting.

One day, at the beginning of our meeting, I asked the questions again, as usual: "Are you still planning to kill yourself?"

"Yes."

"With pills?"

"Yes."

"You have the pills?"

"No."

Confused, I asked, "You don't have the pills?"

"No." She pressed her lips into a determined line.

"What happened to the pills?" I asked.

"I checked, and they had passed their expiration dates, so I threw them away."

I choked back a slight laugh, and then I couldn't help it; I laughed out loud.

"What?" she challenged me, but with a twinkle in her eye and her lips quirking into a grin.

A few seconds later, she burst out laughing with me.

Then she said, "I will begin saving up again, just in case."

NOTES TO THE PRACTITIONER

There are times when the threat of suicide is a call for help or attention, but it is extremely dangerous to underrate the seriousness of any threat of this nature, and it should never be dismissed without further investigation. I repeat: Any mention of suicide should always be regarded with the utmost seriousness.

When evaluating the threat for viability, the first question to ask is "How?" This is in order to understand whether (a) there is a suicide plan, and (b) it's a plan that can in fact be carried out. For example, if the counselee comments, "I'm planning to shoot myself," ask him, "Do you have access to a gun?" If someone wants to jump into a volcano in Hawaii, but does not live in Hawaii and has no plans for getting there, it is not a viable threat.

When the plan *is* viable, the next question is: "When?" If that decision hasn't been made yet, in some cases a trust-based contract can be made, in which the client/patient agrees to tell you if or when such a decision is made. There is some risk involved in this type of contract, but I chose this approach with Harriet, based on both my experience in the field and all the information I received from her during a full hour meeting.

CONCLUSIONS

- *All suicide threats should be taken seriously. If it is unclear whether a suicide threat is real, treat it as if it is.*

- *When checking the level of immediate danger, the existence of a plan, the plan's viability, accessibility to means, and the timing should all be carefully evaluated.*
- *If there is suicide ideation with accessible means, the client or patient should not be allowed to leave the premises without active accomplished referral.*
- *The risk of suicide increases following the receipt of bad news, so a receiver of bad news should not be left unattended.*

RECOMMENDED READING

1. This article focuses on assessment of suicide risk. M. Boldrini and V. Arango, "Stress and Suicide, Conclusions," in *Encyclopedia of Neuroscience* (Amsterdam: Elsevier, 2009), 479. Quoted in *Science Direct*, https://www.sciencedirect.com/topics/medicine-and-dentistry/assessment-of-suicide-risk (accessed August 5, 2021).

2. This significant article focuses on specific factors that should be included in suicide assessment. A very worthwhile read. Thomas H. Valk, "Psychiatric Disorders of Travel, Assessment of Suicide Risk," in *Travel Medicine*, 3rd ed. (Amsterdam: Elsevier, 2013), 447. Quoted in *Science Direct*, https://www.sciencedirect.com/topics/medicine-and-dentistry/assessment-of-suicide-risk (accessed August 5, 2021).

27

✺

Dancing on Blood

The Side Effects of Transplants

Abel lived in a small communal settlement with his wife and three young children. The community pooled its funds for equal distribution, regardless of job title or salary. Every budgetary decision was decided communally, including expenses for housing and renovations. To benefit from that budget, all members waited for their turn according to age, years on the commune, and number of children.

But Abel was waiting for something else: a new heart.

He was scheduled to go to Europe, to wait there for a donor to become available. It was a weird psychological situation. He was going to wait for a healthy person to die, probably in a car crash or some other fatal accident, so that he could receive the victim's heart.

His young wife and three small children would have to wait patiently for him back home. There was no telling how long that wait would be. With any luck, it would only be a month or two; but Judith, Abel's wife, had heard stories of others sometimes waiting years for a heart donor.

Meanwhile, other preparations had to be made. My role was to help them form a plan. My first observation was directed to the heart patient: "You need to renovate your home, Abel."

We were meeting in their living room. It was a small ground-floor apartment with narrow hallways, two small bedrooms, and a single bathroom.

"No, I can't do that," he replied.

Clearing the Path. Lynne Dale Halamish and Eric J. Cassell, Oxford University Press. © Lynne Dale Halamish 2022.
DOI: 10.1093/oso/9780197636879.003.0027

I was insistent. "Abel, when you return with your new heart, things will be different. Your immune system will be compromised. Your body will not be able to effectively fight off illness. You will need to have your own room with a bathroom attached to your house, and a separate entrance."

"I don't see why."

"If one of your kids gets a cold or the flu or anything else, you cannot live in the house with them with a compromised immune system. Not unless you can isolate yourself from germs and viruses the children bring into your house."

"But I can't do that." He looked down miserably at his hands.

"Tell me why," I urged him.

"It's not my turn," he answered plainly.

"Look, Abel." I waited for a moment for his eyes to return to mine before continuing. "If you don't have your own room when you return, you might just as well not get that new heart. You'll die anyway—it's a waste. One day, some minor illness one of your kids brings home will be fatal to you because of your immune system. Don't waste your time and your community's money if you don't plan to take care of yourself after this operation."

He looked appalled. "But you don't understand!"

"Talk to me."

"It would be like I'm using my illness to take something I wouldn't get otherwise. What will everyone think of me? It would be like dancing on blood!"

He was referring to the communal lifestyle, and how important it was to maintain strict equality, without anyone taking unfair advantage or "cutting in line" for benefits. I responded directly to that worry.

"Abel, I guarantee you that no one in your community would be willing to trade places with you in your condition." I leaned in a little further for emphasis. "It's *your own* blood you're talking about."

When it became clear that Abel still didn't feel that he could ask for this special consideration, I asked him for permission to speak to the community leadership on his behalf. As I expected, they readily agreed to prioritize his need; the home renovations took place while he was waiting in Europe. He waited 8 months and was able to return safely to his renovated home with his new heart.

NOTES TO THE PRACTITIONER

As health practitioners, we have expertise that includes outlining a successful recovery plan for a life-threatening condition. In such cases, everyday priorities must be reordered.

We cannot assume that an inexperienced patient will understand the ramifications of their disease, or even of their successful recovery. While the patient and family would like to believe that everything will go back to normal after the crisis passes, the practitioner's responsibility is to look ahead and help them understand and accept the inevitable life changes they will need to make, particularly when not adhering to those changes can be life-threatening.

Long-term preparation may be costly and time-consuming, which makes it even more important to coach the family on how to carry it out.

CONCLUSIONS

- *When dealing with a life-changing situation, priorities must be readjusted.*
- *The practitioner should ensure that the client/patient is aware of as many ramifications, both present and future, as possible.*

RECOMMENDED READING

1. M. Tinetti, L. Dindo, C. D. Smith, C. Blaum, D. Costello, G. Ouellet, J. Rosen, K. Hernandez-Bigos, M. Geda, & A. Naik, "Challenges and Strategies in Patients' Health Priority-Aligned Decision-Making for Older Adults with Multiple Chronic Conditions," *Journal Plos One* (June 10, 2019), https://doi.org/10.1371/journal.pone.0218249 (accessed August 5, 2021).
2. M. Tinetti, A. Naik, L. Dindo, D. Costello, J. Esterson, M. Geda, J. Rosen, K. Hernandez-Bigos, C. D. Smith, G. Ouellet, G. Kang, Y. Lee, and C. Blaum, "Association of Patient Priorities-Aligned Decision-Making with Patient Outcomes and Ambulatory Health Care Burden among Older Adults with Multiple Chronic Conditions: A Nonrandomized Clinical Trial," *JAMA Internal Medicine* 179, no. 12 (October 7, 2019): 1688–1697, https://jamanetwork.com/journals/jamainternalmedicine/fullarticle/2752365 (accessed August 5, 2021).

28

৵৹

Basil

Recovering or Reinventing the Self

The mental health supervisor from the small town came to me and said: "I have someone I would like you to meet. I will completely understand if you refuse. His mother is a permanent resident at our nursing home. He is 27 years old, a real problem in town. He was thrown out of high school for being violent. He was never good in school and is not very bright, he doesn't work well, and he has very few friends. But his father is a good, reliable man, and his brother is wonderful. Would you agree to meet with him? I will completely understand if you refuse."

We had worked together before. But it was the first time she had ever approached me in this way.

"I would be happy to meet with him," I answered. I added a bit doubtfully, "Does *he* want to meet with *me*?"

"We will give him an ultimatum."

"Well," I thought to myself, "this is new. I don't usually get clients by way of threats."

In that short exchange, I had been given a lot of information. It was a family of four: a disabled mother who lived in a nursing home, a "good" father, a "wonderful" brother, and . . . Norman. He was the quintessential "problem child"—violent, angry, stupid, and lazy. Most importantly, his hometown viewed him as a lost cause, who had to be threatened in order to meet with me for his own good. Or perhaps, for the good of the community and family.

Clearing the Path. Lynne Dale Halamish and Eric J. Cassell, Oxford University Press. © Lynne Dale Halamish 2022.
DOI: 10.1093/oso/9780197636879.003.0028

The following week, as I approached the door of his home, I couldn't help but notice that his garden had a large patch of beautiful, healthy basil. It was green, fragrant, and leafy. . . and somehow, this conflicted with the picture of Norman that I had been given.

One of the advantages of meeting patients at their private residence is the information that can be gathered from their "natural habitat." I begin with noting their surroundings—in this instance, it was the garden. The house environment is next. Clean and well lit, or cluttered and dreary? Curtains open or drawn shut? What possessions are left open to view? Then, the individual: What does she or he look like? What is the person wearing? Is there any sign of disability?

Norman came to the door in answer to my knock. He was short and solidly built.

"I noticed you have basil growing in your garden." I looked in admiration at his leafy patch.

"Yes . . ." He avoided my eyes as we spoke.

"It is the most incredible, healthy basil patch I have ever seen. I have tried and tried to grow basil, with no success. How did you do it?"

I stepped back to admire his basil and looked back at him. Clearly, I was waiting to hear his advice on what I needed to change, in order to grow healthy basil. As he explained, he seemed to be standing a little taller than before.

Then we went into the house, and I asked to hear his story.

He described a family with two boys: his brother, the wonderful golden boy; and himself, the horrible, stupid troublemaker who had no control over himself and no future.

His frustration with himself came through his tone and posture, as he confessed, "I am angry *all the time.*"

I thought of the basil patch outside, tended with such patience and discipline, and I found that statement hard to believe. Maybe he was angry most of the time; but it appeared that his home was his haven, his shelter from that storm, where he could forget for a while.

I asked him how long his mother had been in the nursing home, and why she was a permanent resident there. His answer came out in chopped phrases, as though each one hurt while coming out.

"When I was 13 years old, my mother dropped dead. I was in the room with her . . . and I performed CPR on her. It took a long time. But she came around. Only she was severely brain-damaged. That's when she was placed in the nursing home."

"Do you ever see her?"

"I visit her every day."

"Can she talk to you? Does she recognize you?"

His eyes were still fixed on the stone tiles under his feet, as he replied, "Oh yes, she talks to me. She curses me every time I visit. Every single day."

"Does she curse everyone?"

"No, only me."

"Do you know why?"

"For having saved her life."

"Wow!" I exclaimed, "That is possibly the worst story I ever heard. You rescued your mother from death, and instead of being thanked as a hero for such a brave and timely intervention—and who could even believe a 13-year-old could have the presence of mind to do that?—instead, you became the terrible son, the cursed one."

Norman remained silent, his gaze still fixed on the floor tiles.

I thought about this man, who was robbed of his future in one heroic moment, 14 years ago. For him it was over half a lifetime, gone. I felt his anger and pain. I empathized with his loss.

But what could be done about it now? What he had initially experienced as justified anger turned into bitterness during years of being misunderstood. The anger became a habit that pushed others away, and that habit forever cemented his reputation in his village. How could he retrieve something of his potential from this trapped position?

After some moments of silence, I absurdly asked the grown man in front of me: "Norman, what do you want to be when you grow up?"

His answer was both candid and despairing: "I can't do anything. I am too stupid and impulsive."

"Okay." I resisted the urge to disagree with him.

Why? First of all, I didn't know him. Secondly, a stranger's opinion would not effectively change anything—not after years of criticism, reinforced by rejection from everyone around him, backed by his own view of himself.

Instead, I would offer him an escape from that "reality" and a chance to reinvent himself, via a daydreaming exercise.

"Okay, then," I said briskly. "Let's pretend that you could do anything at all—anything you wanted. Knock yourself out. What is your deepest, wildest wish?"

"I want . . . No. I could never."

"Well . . .?"

"Okay. I want . . . a driver's license."

"That's all?"

"Yes, but . . . but, I could never . . ."

"Okay. By the time we meet next week, I want you to get the materials you need to study for the driving theory test."

"But—I am too stupid."

I waved away the comment. "Do you know how many stupid drivers there are? Do you know, for that matter, how many stupid *professors* there are?"

"But I . . ."

"Just get the book. That's your homework assignment."

Norman bought the book and began studying. A month later, he passed the driving theory exam and began taking driving lessons with an instructor. By the end of 3 months, he had his driver's license.

This was the first brick with which we could start to reconstruct a foundation for Norman. We needed a place to rebuild something; or in his case, perhaps to build something for the first time. I could see other places and other bricks that had once been there, but by now they were crushed and unusable. This one brick was whole, and it made a good start.

"Now, Norman, what is your wildest dream, really?"

"To be a medical assistant. But it is a year-long course. I could never do it."

"Sign up."

"But I am too . . ."

"The only stupid thing about you, Norman, is that you *think* you're stupid."

At this point, I still couldn't know that this was true. I wanted it to be true. And from my experience, stupid people rarely tell you that they are stupid. This man was heavily scarred by half a lifetime of incessant criticism. It is difficult to feel through emotional injuries. That's why I chose to be so direct.

"You have already gotten your driver's license. That was the first brick. Now, you will succeed again in this medical assistant's course. A second brick. We will have to build on practical success, progress that you can see for yourself, brick by brick, because you have been brainwashed into believing you can't succeed."

Norman signed up and began the course. I had provided a letter of recommendation to the school for him. I also gave him another assignment:

"I am going to ask you to resist thoughts of 'I can't.' Every time you hear it, I want you to laugh at it, and say out loud, 'Ha! Ridiculous. Of course I can.'"

Repetitive thoughts are usually instilled from childhood. When we hear people attached to a repetitive thought, we can assume that it has been around for over a decade, maybe two. The more it is repeated, the more influential it becomes and usually has to be uprooted. The easiest way to uproot something is to replace it with something else, so that the empty space doesn't become available grounds for resprouting of the old thing.

I have found that it's effective to declare the opposite of the repetitive thought.

Speaking to Norman about this, I added, "It is grueling, slow, painstaking work. You must be vigilant and contradict that 'I can't' thought whenever it resurfaces."

"But I really don't believe that I *can*."

"You don't have to believe it. For the time being, I will believe it for you. Just say it. Out loud. Make it go out of your mouth and in through your ears."

It was now time to deal with Norman's mother and her cursing. While trying to rebuild his fragile ego, Norman cannot have it torn down again every time he visits his mom, who keeps proclaiming him a failure. He also cannot stop visiting her, because this, too, would make him feel like an unworthy son. Yet he cannot make her change. Or, can he?

How did his dilemma take shape in the first place?

Norman had been marked at age 13 by a trauma. He had performed a resuscitation on his own mother that was remarkably heroic and quick-thinking; it was successful, yet it had disastrous consequences. The repercussions of that mixed result were felt communally as well as in his family. But what of the repercussions on the boy-rescuer himself? Hadn't Norman been deprived of any chance for a normal life?

Can such a loss be recovered through intervention? The short answer is, "Maybe." Therefore, it is always worth trying.

Over all those years, Norman and his mother had developed a dynamic, a dance. In this dance, they each have a part. Let's say the dance is a rumba. If he begins to dance the cha-cha, she can no longer "rumba" with him. The pattern is disrupted, and the interaction must change.

"You visit her every day?"

"Yes."

"Why?"

"Because she's my mother."

"How do you feel when she curses you?"

"Angry and ashamed."

"Norman, she is battering you, beating you up every time you go there. She is brain-damaged, but she is able to communicate, so perhaps she's aware of what she's doing. Do not let her treat you this way."

"But it's my fault."

I didn't try to argue with him. I paused for a moment, to gather my thoughts.

"When you visit her today, sit down and tell her that you will not listen to her cursing anymore. That if she curses you, you will leave."

"What will happen then?"

"She will curse you, and you will get up and leave. Go see her again the next day. But the first time she curses you, get up and walk out. She will eventually get it, and if she wants to have visitors—and you are almost the only one who visits—she will eventually stop."

He began to follow this instruction. Within a few weeks, the cursing had almost stopped. But it had been replaced by silence and baleful looks.

"What should I do now?" he asked me.

"Tell her about your dreams for the future. Tell her what you are doing now. If she starts to laugh at you or tell you that you can't succeed, get up and leave. Do this until she can listen to what you say without making you feel bad."

Our meetings ended there.

Thirteen years passed.

I was walking one day through the same small town, on my way to see another client, when suddenly I was nearly tackled by a man who ran to me and hugged me, exclaiming, "Lynne, Lynne, Lynne!"

I stepped back out of the hug, a little off-balance, and looked up at the excited man, not recognizing him at all.

"Lynne, I'm so happy to see you. You saved my life!"

"Remind me . . .?" I asked, bewildered.

"It's me, Norman!" he replied. He then gave me a summary of our meetings together.

"Oh, Norman!" I took his hand warmly in both of mine. "How are you?"

"I'm great!" he announced, beaming. "I have a new career, I'm married, and I have three wonderful children. I've even become accepted and respected in my community, all thanks to you!"

I smiled broadly but refused the praise. "No, Norman. Not at all. *You* did the work. I was just your witness."

NOTES TO THE PRACTITIONER

In this case, it was important to pay attention to the patient's physical surroundings, in order to gain additional first-hand information. Before actually meeting this client, I could have been strongly biased against him due to the "information" I was given during the referral. Seeing his garden prompted me to question what I had been told.

Once a "label" is assigned to a patient in a ward, or to a client in a community, it is quite difficult to see the person behind the tag. As it turned out, I saw no indication that Norman was "a real problem, not bright, or doesn't work well" during the entire time I worked with him.

When he told me his story, my reaction ("That is possibly the worst thing I ever heard") was spontaneous and honest. This support, which was recognition of the injustice he had endured, encouraged him to trust me.

When patients belittle themselves to you, do not contradict them unless (until) you have tangible evidence to the contrary. It is a much more effective tool to use doable tasks to assist them in building their self-worth. When they accomplish these tasks, encourage them by giving them full credit for the work they have done.

CONCLUSIONS

- *Pay attention to the patient's natural habitat. It can give you a lot of information.*
- *Recurring thoughts are usually instilled at a young age. One way to combat those thoughts is to repudiate them, out loud.*
- *Practical tasks undertaken successfully may provide proof to refute ceaseless negative thoughts and improve self-image.*

RECOMMENDED READING

1. Joaquín Selva, "5 Worksheets for Challenging Negative Automatic Thoughts," *Positive Psychology* (October 13, 2020), https://positivepsychology.com/challenging-automatic-thoughts-positive-thoughts-worksheets/ (accessed August 5, 2021).
2. Rebecca Joy Stanborough, "How to Change Negative Thinking with Cognitive Restructuring: Techniques and Examples," *Healthline* (February 4, 2020), https://www.healthline.com/health/cognitive-restructuring (accessed August 5, 2021).

29

⁂

The Stuff of Dreams

Finding the Meaning

I was counseling a bereaved family immediately after a death. The family consisted of the mother Becky, her husband, and their four children. There had originally been five children, but the 14-year-old daughter and sister, Shelly, had taken a public bus home from school and had been killed by a suicide bomber, along with several other victims.

I met the entire family a few times, and later I had individual meetings with the parents and each of the children for about a year. However, I continued to periodically meet with Becky for several years, at her request.

Five and a half years after Shelly's death, Becky wrote me a letter, telling me about a particular dream she had had. She simply couldn't shake it off. She reviewed it, trying to make sense of it, but to no avail. She asked to see me about it.

As she began to describe the dream to me, she spoke slowly. "I was taking an afternoon nap in full sunlight on our bed. I was feeling worn out, and I was enjoying the sun's warmth as I drifted off to sleep. I had a dream. . . . It was striking and vivid but also deeply confusing. It had a chain of events that I could follow, but at one point I was startled awake by the phone ringing. I have no idea what to make of it. It seemed significant. I was sure it was a bad omen."

I leaned toward her slightly. "Go on," I urged.

"In the dream, I'm walking down the street. I glance at my own reflection in a store window and I notice a wound on my head. I step closer to the

Clearing the Path. Lynne Dale Halamish and Eric J. Cassell, Oxford University Press. © Lynne Dale Halamish 2022.
DOI: 10.1093/oso/9780197636879.003.0029

glass and say to myself, 'I thought I took care of that before . . .' and I look more closely at it. It's a big, open wound. I'm startled by it, and I reach up and touch it, and—up from the wound comes a big sac of pus. It starts oozing. I'm repulsed and horrified as I touch it, and it pops open."

"Suddenly, from that big, open wound, out pops this beautiful orchid. I don't even like orchids, but this one was particularly stunning. I think to myself, 'That's weird,' and I pull on it a bit—and two more flowers pop out on this vine. I pull some more, and eight or nine new flowers appear. 'I shouldn't pull on it anymore. I need to see a doctor,' I say to myself aloud in the dream."

"So, I go to my husband and say, 'I need a doctor, I don't understand, this shouldn't be growing out of my head!' But he isn't looking; his eyes are fixed on his work. I demand, 'Look at me!'"

"He finally looks up at me and says, 'Oh, that's really beautiful.'"

"I look back at him and ask, 'Are you joking?! I have a *plant* growing out of my *head!*'"

"That's when the phone rang and woke me up."

I suggested to Becky that perhaps we could try to interpret the dream together. The interpretation method I prefer is based on the hypothesis that everyone and everything in the dream is part of the dreamer. So, to find the dream's meaning, the dreamer reviews the dream repeatedly, each time from the perspective of one of the characters or objects in the dream. During each review, I ask questions for clarification.

We began with the store window, treating it as a thinking being. The window observes the woman looking into it and seeing the wound, then the pus, then the flowers, and panicking. Becky put the window's thoughts into words: "I see it all from the outside."

Then she responded to questions taking the part of the wound: It hurts the woman by building up pressure, but it needs to come out. After the flowers pop out, the pressure is somewhat eased, but not gone. "I (the wound) want her (the woman) to leave me alone."

After that, Becky took the part of the pus coming out of the head wound. I asked: "Are you inside Becky's skull, or on the outside?"

The answer was more hesitant. "I don't know . . . Inside. No. No, outside. No, wait—inside. Yes. I am inside Becky's head."

"How long have you been there?" I continued to ask.

"I've been in there for a lifetime. But I began to grow 5 years ago."

"Are you weak or strong?"

Becky answered without hesitation: "Strong enough to break hard ground."

A new clue. I looked at her intently. "Do you have another name, other than 'sac of pus'?"

Becky paused. Her eyes momentarily narrowed and moved to the side, then back to meet mine. "I am not a pus sac." Her eyes became blurred by a wall of tears. "I am a seed."

"This is good," I encouraged her. "A seed is a more solid thing. Does the seed have a name?"

Becky's voice became small and distant. "There is a name, but I can't hear it."

"You say it's been there all your life. Who planted the seed before you were born?"

Becky paused again and then spoke. "God," she said, and she wept.

"Listen carefully," I said quietly. "What is the name of the seed? Listen to the voice that is telling you its name."

"I hear 'Wisdom'. . . I hear it, but I don't believe." Her weeping continued.

"Describe wisdom to me."

"Wisdom is seeing the truth and applying it."

"What else?"

"It begins with God."

I urged her to dig deeper. "What else?"

Becky continued, "It is precious. It is not listened to. It is valuable."

"Like an orchid?" I asked.

"Yes." Her eyebrows raised in realization.

"And?" I sensed that there was more. "What else?"

Again her eyes narrowed, as she looked to the side, then widened as her eyes again met mine. "Wisdom is a woman."

"Yes. This is very powerful. Becky, listen. Your name is not 'pus sac'. Your name is 'wisdom'. This is something that everyone can see, except for you."

Becky looked at me attentively as I went on: "Pay attention. In your dream, your husband told you that the flowers were beautiful. In your dream, you knew that there were more orchids still in your head. You stopped pulling only because you thought it shouldn't be happening."

Becky had let go and was crying freely.

This was a transformative dream. I felt it then and there, in the meeting. But that was 2008.

While writing this book (2021), I decided to see if it was truly transformative for the dreamer. I called Becky to hear how she was doing. Would she even remember the dream?

Becky answered immediately. "Oh yes, I remember very well. It was indeed significant."

"In what way?" I asked.

"The dream, and your questions about it, sent me on a transformative journey. This seed that God planted within me is part of who I am, a core part of myself. But at the time I wasn't aware of it. Uncovering that piece of me allowed me to begin being who I am, without being bound by fear."

She continued: "The orchids are the fruit of my journey. It's a peaceful and beautiful journey. It doesn't need to compete for attention or struggle to find its place. It *has* a place. This journey has included dismantling a false self that was created to fulfill my own expectations, as well as those of others around me."

"The dream, and the analysis we did that day, have accompanied me through all the years since then. Our family's collective and individual journey through grief has been very long . . . and at times, very dark. The dream, and my understanding of it, gave me hope both for myself and my family."

> Deep in your wounds are seeds,
> Waiting to grow beautiful flowers.
>
> —Niti Majethia

NOTES TO THE PRACTITIONER

I rarely explore dreams with clients, because of the fluid nature of dreams and their interpretations. It can even be a manipulative process if misapplied. But occasionally, getting to the bottom of a significant dream can jump-start a person's way to recovery.

Dreams are triggered by many things, and they can sometimes reveal secrets that we cannot or will not discover during our waking, conscious hours. How can you as a practitioner know a dream might be significant? Usually, the main sign is when it stays with the dreamer, when they cannot let it go, when it intrudes into their thoughts repeatedly. Another sign is a dream that keeps returning. The repetition is sometimes an indication of its significance.

A transformative experience changes you or the path you are on in a significant way. What is a transformative dream? It's one that can generate change, growth, or action. Perhaps your unconscious is telling you something that you cannot hear through any other means.

Becky's dream was transformative. I felt that in the meeting, by remaining attentive to her reactions to it. With transformative dreams, uncovering the meaning behind them can allow the dreamer to apply the transformation to their life, briefly recognize it, or ignore it. This type of dream can have great value when understood and applied.

In Becky's case, she realized that the "wisdom seed" was always there, but it only began to grow following the traumatic death of her daughter. Thus, we see that even trauma can have a benefit, despite the unspeakable price.

CONCLUSIONS

- *Even trauma or loss can be a turning point in life for benefit or realizing new potential.*
- *Sometimes, while treating a patient or client, we will be handed a "gift" like a dream, which provides both dreamer and counselor with additional tools to assist them.*
- *When a dying patient dreams of a reunion with a deceased family member, it may be time to call the family in to say goodbye. In my experience, it usually means that death is very close.*

RECOMMENDED READING

1. Brenda Mallon, *Dying, Death and Grief: Working with Adult Bereavement* (Los Angeles: SAGE, 2008), 120.
2. Margret Wilkinson, "The Dreaming Mind-Brain: A Jungian Perspective," *Journal of Analytical Psychology* 51, no. 1 (February 2006): 43–59, https://pubmed.ncbi. nlm.nih.gov/16451317 (accessed August 5, 2021).

30

ᴄⱱᴐ

Surviving Death

The End of Grief

Can grief end?
Here is my story.
Since Zohar had been killed, happiness and joy were not a part of our family repertoire. Zohar, my husband Asaf's biological son, and my son by marriage from age 6, was an IDF artillery officer. He was shot and killed in battle 2 months after his 21st birthday.

Five years later, Asaf attended a communications seminar from work. He seemed different.

A few days after the seminar, Asaf came to me excitedly. "Lynnie—look, the sparkle has come back to my eyes!"

"What?" I replied. "What are you talking about?"

"The sparkle! I haven't seen it for 5 years, and today I looked in the mirror . . . and it's back."

I looked at him. It *was* back. What was this?

"Talk to me," I said.

Then Asaf began to describe his journey to me. "You know, I went to a three-day communications seminar. They said, 'Ask for any three things you want, possible or not.' I said: 'I want my own start-up R&D company where all employees are creative, writing on the floor, the walls, a never-ending brainstorm. I want two million dollars in the bank. And I want my dead son back.'"

Clearing the Path. Lynne Dale Halamish and Eric J. Cassell, Oxford University Press. © Lynne Dale Halamish 2022.
DOI: 10.1093/oso/9780197636879.003.0030

Asaf looked down at his hands and then to a spot somewhere over my shoulder. He slowly began to speak again.

"At some point, I realized that I had been building walls ever since we lost Zohar. Walls around walls, and more walls around those walls around myself, so that nothing could ever touch me again. Walls that kept out any sliver of light and kept me in complete, solitary darkness. Brick by brick, my fortress became my prison, and I continued fortifying it for 5 long years."

"What did that darkness look like?" I asked.

"Loss of joy, laughter, fun family time, personal freedom. I was a walking dead man, for 5 years. The walls had locked me out of life. The constant grief, anger, and longing left no cracks for any life to shine through."

"On the one hand, I was grasping at any pieces left of Zohar: his pictures, his friends—and if not them, his possessions, his clothing, his journals, and even grief itself. On the other hand, I felt I had to protect myself from being too close to our children, to you, or anyone else I held dear. I was unaware this was happening at the time. I only became aware of this after the walls finally fell."

He let out one long exhale that made his cheeks flare slightly, before speaking again.

"But as it turned out, I built these walls out of my fear of going through another unbearable loss. If I could just refrain from ever loving anyone that much again, I could prevent that searing pain. I knew there was no way we . . . I . . . could ever live through that twice."

He leaned forward and reached for the cup of tea on the wooden table in front of us, then leaned back, cupping it in his hands.

"As the years went by, I wasn't even able to see Zohar clearly in my mind anymore; all I could see was death and darkness wherever I looked. Not only were my walls keeping out my loved ones, they were keeping my son's memory in complete darkness, too. There was this one moment during the seminar when I suddenly realized that what I had been building was not a haven at all. I had imprisoned myself in a dungeon. The seminar helped me see that I was fooling myself with the illusion of safety and control. This realization allowed me to finally let go, knock the walls down, and break out. That's how I reclaimed the life I lost 5 years ago."

Asaf's eyes wandered as a small hummingbird hovered near the sugared feeder outside our living room window. The wrinkles in the corner of his eyes deepened as he smiled at it for a moment. And again, I saw the "sparkle" that he had been talking about.

Asaf had returned to the family. He was suddenly involved and interested in everything again. He convinced me to also try this communications seminar.

I was skeptical.

But I went.

I encountered 30-odd people and an arrogant (albeit charismatic) "group facilitator," all sitting in a circle. I hated this kind of stuff. They tell you to talk to your neighbor, and then *you* have to introduce *that guy* to the entire group. I am *not* interested in my neighbor. I will never even remember his name—let alone all the other crap he deems important to share with me.

Oh great: Now the facilitator is introducing himself. He thinks he's funny. So does this group of lawyers, army officers, police, medical and mental health practitioners, and others.

Since Zohar's death, the simplest questions have become the hardest ones: "How many people are in your family?" "How many kids do you have?" "How old is your eldest?" Damned if you answer, damned if you don't.

Now it's almost my turn. I do *not* want to do this. My heart is racing, and I can feel my face turning red.

All eyes turned to me as I began to speak: "My name is Lynne Halamish. I am married and have four kids. One is dead."

Just as the words left my mouth, I burst into tears and couldn't stop crying! *Oh no! I have to spend 3 days with these people!*

Everyone looked anxious, except for the facilitator, may his name and memory be erased. He told everyone to settle down and asked the next person to introduce himself. He did. I was still sniffling and snorting as the introductions continued, trying to regain composure. *How did this happen? I am usually so in control.*

Suddenly the facilitator turned to me and shot a question in my direction. "Do you trust me?" he asked.

"I don't trust anyone," I replied.

"When did you stop trusting anyone?" he asked.

"May 18, 1993." The reply flew out from between my lips before I could think. The day my son was killed. This was a revelation. I had never connected my distrust of others with Zohar's death before.

A few hours later, or maybe it was even the next day, the facilitator led us in a guided imagery session. We were asked to imagine ourselves walking into our family room. I was overwhelmed with surprise and joy to find my family whole, safe, and happy in my mind. My four beautiful children were all there.

Somehow, Zohar was back in my life.

I could reflect on all of our shared memories throughout the years with joy, laughter, and sometimes regret—for what I hadn't had the chance to do with him in the past and what I would never get to do with him in the future. After years of being clouded by mourning, I could finally see him again.

It was like coming out of the cold, where even breathing is difficult. And then, one day, you suddenly take a deep breath and realize your lungs are full of air again.

Two days later, we were in a circle again. People are sharing experiences. I want to reintroduce myself. So, I do:

"My name is Lynne Halamish. I am a thanatologist. I am married to Asaf, a wonderful man, my best friend, support, and lover. I have four wonderful children. Shachar, 14, is deep and considerate. Hilah, 11, is quick-witted and wise. Oriah, 8, is affectionate and generous. And Zohar, my eldest, is intelligent and sensitive."

"I still have Asaf, Shachar, Hilah, and Oriah; I don't know for how long. I had Zohar for 15 years. I won't have him anymore, but I won't have him any less either."

Everyone in the circle is in tears—except me.

So, can grief end?

Yes. Grief can end.

But the end of grief does not mean erasing or forgetting the deceased. It means tearing down the wall of grief so you can "see" them again. (For a more detailed explanation, go to Appendix B, "Looking for the End of Grief.")

How do I know this? How could I? Has it been verified empirically?

The main reason I know this is that I've been down that path, following my own stepson's death. Yes, this story is my story, and this grief has reached its end.

As an experienced professional, this of course was not enough to prove that grief could end; there are many variables. My husband has trod this path, along with and separately from me, and he has seen the end of grief. Asaf and I both reached our personal end of grief about 5 years after our eldest son's sudden death.

Once I knew it was possible, I had the privilege of helping many clients through this process and witnessing the end of their grief over children, parents, siblings, spouses. Whether illness, injury, accident, war, suicide, or murder had taken their loved ones from them, or whether they were grieving over the loss of a physical part of themselves—I have seen it, time and time again:

All grief has a beginning, a middle, and a possible end.

NOTES TO THE PRACTITIONER

We know from general observation, backed by research, that grief can end. We may even expect it to end within a ridiculously short period of time, which is not consistent with reality. At the other extreme, however, is a kind of grief that is expected to *never* end; and that is the message often given to parents who have lost a child.

This is an understandable assumption. Unlike "natural order" family deaths (grandparents before parents, parents before children, etc.), children dying before their parents or grandparents is considered "unnatural." It's a premature loss that stretches far into the future.

Even with "natural" death, the end of grief is frequently obstructed and prolonged by public opinion, guilt, or a sense of obligation that makes grieving an ingrained habit. A child's death brings all these difficulties, while simultaneously destroying any naivete regarding death being predictable.

Two of the most common responses of bereaved parents are *abandonment* or *suffocation*. In the first case, the parent creates emotional distance from their remaining children, to try to protect themselves. In the second, they overly interfere or interject themselves into the remaining children's lives, in an effort to protect them. It is more common for the father to abandon, and for the mother to suffocate the surviving children. It is uncommon to see both parents with the same response; usually one parent responds one way, and the other parent will respond the other way.

Finding the end of this grief path requires internalizing a truth, which is not as simple as it sounds: Every griever has a right, even an obligation, to live and not just to exist. One's life is meant to be more than a memorial to the dead.

CONCLUSIONS

- *Despite beliefs to the contrary, grief for a deceased child is like every other grief: it has a beginning, a middle, and a potential end.*
- *When such grief does not end, it is worth examining whether the parent knows that it can end and/or requires "permission" to live rather than just exist.*
- *Ending grief is not an erasure or betrayal of the deceased. It does not mean you didn't and don't still love and miss them.*

RECOMMENDED READING

1. "Understanding When Grief Is Complete," *MentalHelp Net*, https://www.men
   talhelp.net/grief-and-bereavement/understanding-when-grief-is-complete
   (accessed August 5, 2021).
2. Sherry Cormier, "Will My Grief Ever End? Here's How You Can Grieve Well and
   Help Yourself through the Painful Process," *ThriveWorks Counseling* (September
   4, 2018), https://thriveworks.com/blog/grieve-well-help-yourself-painful-proc
   ess (accessed August 5, 2021).

APPENDIX A

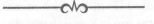

The Toolbox

THINGS THAT CAN MAKE A DIFFERENCE

This chapter is a collection of information accumulated from years of working in the field.

Help along the Path

Following are some practical tips from people whom I have counseled, which they have generously agreed to share. These are coping strategies that other grievers may find helpful.

Widowhood

- Put a hot water bottle in bed 10 minutes before you go to sleep at night. It is hard to get into a cold bed when you are not used to it.
- Getting a professional massage can sometimes help if you are the kind of person who enjoys being massaged. The lack of touch is a problem in widowhood. A word of warning: Do not be alarmed if you begin to cry when the massage begins. It is normal, and it may even help.

- If your loved one died from an illness, remove all traces of the disease from your living space, like medications and any medical equipment. They are symbols of suffering, pain, and sickness; they are *not* symbols of the person you lost.
- On your first significant holiday after being widowed, don't ignore the absence of your loved one. Instead, point to it explicitly, so that everyone can begin to breathe a little. You can do this by making a toast to "those who could not be here today." You can ask a family member to prepare a story about the deceased loved one, not necessarily a grief story, but a life story, even a funny one to remember at the table. This meal will be peppered with sighs, tears, and laughter. All are fine, and it helps to let a little emotion out.

Bereaved Families

- Sometimes adopting a pet can be helpful. Pets provide unadorned affection, and more particularly, they soften the blow of coming home to an empty house. Bringing a dog into the family can provide additional benefits, such as daily exercise and social interactions with other dog owners. Adopting a pet also helps bereaved siblings, who sometimes find it helpful to confide their fears and secrets to their nonjudgmental furry friend.
- If a parent is bereaved of a school-aged child, the first day of school is a minefield. It will be hard to see other children in the neighborhood, or even other children in the same family, preparing and going to school. Knowing that ahead of time can be helpful.
- Sometimes, well-meaning friends invite bereaved parents to the weddings of their deceased son's or daughter's friends. These events can be real challenges, highlighting their consciousness of loss to include no marriage for their dead child and no grandchildren from them. This invitation can be legitimately refused; however, if the bereaved parents desire or feel obligated to attend a wedding or birth-related celebration, it's best that they attend the ceremony and leave immediately afterwards. Congratulate the couple ahead of time, or as soon after the ceremony as possible, and then, having fulfilled your obligation, just leave. Understand that it will likely be difficult.

Children Who Have Lost a Sibling

- Children are usually the abandoned grievers. Always treat them as part of the family.
- Don't tell them to be strong, and don't allow them to think they must replace the dead child.
- When they ask questions, refer the questions back to them, to hear what they think and believe. Then, give them clear answers to their inquiries, with as much detail as possible. It may seem scary to talk about death with children, but the unknown is far more frightening.

Help to Start the Path: Advice for Practitioners

First Moments after Death: Care for the Body

The deceased was your patient. Before the family comes back into the room to say goodbye, try to wash the face or mouth and straighten the body before the muscles stiffen. Turn on the air conditioner and cover the body with a sheet, leaving the face uncovered. If the body is disfigured in some way, reduce the lighting in the room to make it less stark.

The family decides when they have had enough time to say goodbye, although some gentle guidance from the staff may be needed when the body starts discoloring. Up to 3 hours is okay, and most people don't stay longer than a few minutes.

WHAT TO DO NEXT: Just be there.

The family has entered an entirely new reality. Even if they had advance notice, there is no way to be prepared for death. Stay in the room, unless you feel that the family wants you to leave. If you think this, *ask them* if they would like you to step out of the room. If they say yes, let them know you will be right outside the door if they need you. If you are in a hospital or institution, don't leave before they do.

WHAT TO SAY: As little as possible.

Frequently the family will wait for confirmation that the family member has died. A professional saying, "It's over," may signal the time for crying or screaming or expressing emotions. This is good. Do not try to stop their show of emotions or calm them down. It is important for them to do this their way, not your way. You don't have to say much. When words have no purpose, silence is best.

"Blessed is the man who, having nothing to say, abstains from giving us wordy evidence of the fact." — George Eliot.

WHAT *NOT* TO SAY: Most of the typical "comfort" lines.

Do not say, "S/he is not suffering anymore;" or "It's for the best" (although it's fine if the family says that). Again, your best tool is usually silence. If it is appropriate *and true*, after about 10 minutes of silence, you can say, "S/he looks so peaceful." This will help them to remember their loved one looking peaceful. This is especially important in cases that involved a great deal of pain and suffering near the end.

TO HUG OR NOT TO HUG: It depends.

The question of whether or not you should offer a condolence hug to someone depends on two things: you and them. If you don't feel comfortable hugging, don't do it. It will turn into an awkward moment and make you both uncomfortable. If they exhibit any reluctance (not meeting your gaze, pulling or leaning back, "guarding" their body with their arms or an object), don't do it. A hand on the shoulder is plenty of physical contact to many people.

HOW ELSE YOU CAN HELP: Your presence and attention are valuable.

This is a time for being, more than doing. Pay attention to the family. Make yourself available to them, not only physically but consciously. Look them in the eyes and give them the time, support, and respect they need from you. Talking is the "work" of mourning for most people. Be willing to answer any questions, and listen without contradicting or interrupting (unless you feel they are becoming dangerous to you, to someone else, or to themselves).

Later, possibly at the formal mourning ceremonies if you decide to attend, give the family any stories about the deceased that could make them happy. Present them with any relevant photos or drawings, and repeat any expression of love that you heard . . . even if they heard it, too. They need to be reminded that the deceased cared for them, if indeed that was the case. These expressions are not limited to words; they can also be observations like "I saw the way he looked at you when you . . ." Only stay faithful to the truth.

APPENDIX B

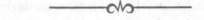

Looking for the End of Grief

During my practice as a thanatologist for over three decades, I discovered a reality that contradicts popular belief: Grief is not a place or a condition; it's a path. It has a beginning, a middle, and a possible end. This is true for all grief.

I hesitate to use the word *all*. Has it been verified empirically that even difficult grief has an end? Well, yes. I traveled that difficult path following my stepson's death, and I reached its end. My husband also walked that path, partly along with me and at times separately from me, and he has also seen the end of grief. (See Chapter 30 for our story.)

As professionals, of course, this is not enough to prove that grief can end. There are many variables to consider. But once I knew it was possible, I had the privilege of helping many clients through this process and witnessing the end of their grief over the loss of children, parents, siblings, and spouses. The circumstances have likewise been varied: whether it was illness, injury, accident, war, suicide, or murder that took their loved ones from them—or even mourning over the loss of a physical part of themselves—I have seen it, time and time again. Grief can end.

LEVELS OF DIFFICULTY IN GRIEVING

How long is the path of grieving? We usually measure it in time. In cases of "natural order" deaths (grandparents before parents, parents before children, etc.), we usually witness a gradual diminishment of sorrow, grief, and pain within 1–2 years following the loss.

With bereavement that causes a change in status (widowhood, bereavement of an only child, or orphanhood through the loss of both parents), or is in "the wrong order" (child before parent), or involves intent (suicide or murder), grief can also end, although it is more complicated and more difficult to predict when it can end.

However, not everyone finds the end.

These paths are frequently obstructed by public opinion, guilt, and/or cultural taboos surrounding a particular kind of death. Grief can last so long that it becomes a habit, and then the habit must also break in order for the grief to end. Many times, the griever doesn't even know that the option of ending the grief exists.

These obstructions in turn are rooted in the most common obstacle of all: ignorance about what the healthy grieving process is like.

WHAT GRIEVING IS AND ISN'T

After the death of a significant other, what does the grief feel like? The only description that I can give is my own experience both personally and in the field: There is no sunshine, no color, and no joy in your life.

What does the end of grief look and feel like? The sunshine, color, and level of joy return. (This is provided that you had joy before the loss. You won't get back what you didn't lose.) You find that you can focus beyond your loss of the loved one, and the memory of their life and their interactions with you brings you joy.

Our dead continue to live in our memory. That is, they exist historically, aside from personal faith-related questions about an afterlife. In this form the person remains with the griever, who reenacts, regurgitates, and relives remembered life events, gradually distorting them in one way or another, removing them from their original context and emotional impact.

This glimpse of the path's end was eloquently described by the British writer-philosopher C. S. Lewis, who had lost his wife to cancer:

> And suddenly at the very moment when, so far, I mourned H. least, I remembered her best. Indeed it was something (almost) better than memory; an instantaneous, unanswerable impression. To say it was like a meeting would be going too far. Yet there was that in it which tempts one to use those words. It was as if the lifting of the sorrow removed a barrier ... For, as I have discovered, passionate grief does not link us with the dead but cuts us off from them. (*A Grief Observed*, 1961)

From this, we can conclude what ending grief does NOT mean:

- It is NOT erasing the deceased.
- It is NOT forgetting them.
- It does NOT mean you didn't and don't love them.
- It does NOT mean you don't miss them.

Lewis discovered this in his own grieving process, and he was chagrined at his previous ignorance:

> Why has no one told me these things? How easily I might have misjudged another man in the same situation? I might have said, "He's got over it. He's forgotten his wife," when the truth was, "He remembers her better because he has partly got over it." (*A Grief Observed*, 1961)

Moreover, engaging in life—working, socializing, and forming new relationships—should all happen *while grieving*, and not wait until afterwards. Fighting to live, and not merely exist, is part of walking the path.

In that fight to live, neither the intensity of grief nor its end can be measured by the griever's activity level. Throughout the decades of doing what I do, I have found almost no connection between grief and functioning. The efficient hard worker is always an efficient hard worker, grieving or not. The inefficient, idle person is always an inefficient, idle person, only with a better excuse as a griever. This is a personality component, and we are often deceived into thinking that the more driven, functioning people must have finished grieving. For them, however, work is frequently a means to escape from grieving or to freeze the grief. Either way, functionality is not a good indicator.

Neither is the quite common tendency of people during grief to "drift" back and forth between faith in God and atheism. This is because when death is the outcome, no answer seems adequate. The griever's spiritual state at the path's end usually depends on the depth of their rooted belief in either side. The grievers with deep roots, after a struggle, generally return to their original convictions.

CLEARING THE PATH: THE ESSENTIALS

So, how can we smooth the path from loss to life, and not merely existence, for these grievers? The first essential is *a separation between the grief and the deceased*. Often, grievers fear letting go of their feelings of loss and sadness because they feel like they would be letting go of the person they lost. It needs to be made clear that grief is 100% *not* the deceased person. We know this because the grief only comes to us immediately after we find out that our loved one has left us. If holding onto the grief is not holding onto the deceased, then there is no reason to hold it longer than necessary.

There are reasons to bring grief to an end. One thing needs to be understood, which is no simple thing: *The griever has a right, even an obligation, to live.* Not just to exist. Each person's life is meant to be more than merely a memorial for the dead, no matter how much we miss them. After all, the griever's life is also finite and will someday end. No life should be ignored or diminished for the sake of the memory of another life that has already ended.

This list summarizes the typical traps that may block someone from reaching the end of their grief process:

1. Grasping

The mistaken notion that holding onto the grief is another way of holding onto the deceased—and if you let it go, you lose them forever.

2. Guilt

The feeling, particularly among bereaved parents, that the death of their child is their fault, and/or they no longer deserve to live once their son or daughter has died.

3. No Permission

The myth that grief over a premature death is never-ending, so the griever doesn't know that it is possible, or even permissible, to ever stop grieving.

4. Ambivalence

Grief over a person who abused the griever. This can be mixed with a feeling of release and even joy over the death of the abuser, which can generate confusion or guilt.

5. Habit

The griever grieves for so long that it becomes a habit that is difficult to break.

6. Misuse of Memorials

The notion that memorials are for the dead, and therefore they cannot be discontinued without betraying or abandoning the deceased loved one. The grief expressed in a memorial is for the griever, not for the dead.

7. Disbelief

Olympic runners periodically break speed records known as "a glass ceiling," because they reject the prevailing belief that there is no way past that invisible barrier. Interestingly, once the barrier is broken, other runners in future Olympic games will surpass even that "impossible" record. The psychological barrier to finishing grief functions in a similar way. For those who don't believe it is possible, it isn't.

8. Status/Secondary Benefit

When there is a secondary benefit derived from remaining a griever, such as the status of being the widow of an important person, or a monetary benefit. Sometimes this is an incentive for a griever to retain this status, regardless of the heavy price to be paid.

THE SUDDENNESS OF GRIEF'S END

Grief is a long process taking several years. It takes a long time to reach the point when grief can potentially end. But once that point is reached, many times the grief will end without warning, surprisingly, instantaneously.

It seems that ending grief requires a trigger. The catalyst can be almost anything: a flash of inner realization, a form of therapy, learning a new skill like chocolate-making, or starting a new direction in life.

There is a way for each griever to find the end of the grief path, and it may likely be tailored according to who they are. Once they know that the end is somewhere up ahead, they can more easily recognize it.

AFTERWORD

Isn't that just like a book on death and dying, an afterward.

During the writing of *Clearing the Path: On Death, Grief, and Loss*, shortly after the final manuscript was delivered to the publisher, my dear friend and writing and teaching mentor, Eric J. Cassell, died shortly after his 93rd birthday.

Eric was a wonderful, astute, and generous man with a mind like a razor and a tongue to match. Psshh. It was such a privilege to know him.

I met him when he came to speak at the Technion, over a decade and a half earlier. I was the local talent and Eric was the amazing, funny star attraction from New York.

Two or three years later, I began to write what became *The Weeping Willow*. After I had written three stories, I wondered if they were worth anything and in order to find out, I decided to find Eric and ask him. I found his contact details, sent him a letter with the three stories, and asked him to comment if he had time, and if not, to continue to "wow" his readers and his audiences.

He didn't remember our previous meeting, but he really liked the stories.

Thus began our amazing connection. He was a precise surgeon of words, the perfect mentor. No fluff, just clear wisdom and truth.

He was a great blessing to me and still is, because the things he taught me are part of who I have become professionally and personally.

It is difficult to put into words how significant Eric has been in my life's journey.

May his name and memory be blessed and continue to bless.